Workbook for
Hartman's Nursing Assistant Care
Long-Term Care

By Hartman Publishing, Inc.

SECOND EDITION

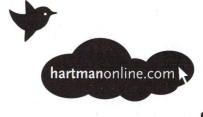

hartmanonline.com

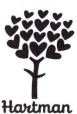

Hartman

ii

Credits

Managing Editor
Susan Alvare Hedman

Cover Designer
Kirsten Browne

Cover Illustrator
Jo Tronc

Interior Designer
Thaddeus Castillo

Interior Illustrator
Thaddeus Castillo

Composition
Thaddeus Castillo
Dara Elerath

Proofreaders
Kristin Calderon
Dara Elerath
Rachel Miller

Copyright Information

Notice to Readers

Though the guidelines and procedures contained in this text are based on consultations with healthcare professionals, they should not be considered absolute recommendations. The instructor and readers should follow employer, local, state, and federal guidelines concerning healthcare practices. These guidelines change, and it is the reader's responsibility to be aware of these changes and of the policies and procedures of her or his healthcare facility.

The publisher, author, editors, and reviewers cannot accept any responsibility for errors or omissions or for any consequences from application of the information in this book and make no warranty, expressed or implied, with respect to the contents of the book. The publisher does not warrant or guarantee any of the products described herein or perform any analysis in connection with any of the product information contained herein.

Table of Contents

Preface

Welcome to the *Workbook for Nursing Assistant Care: Long-Term Care*! This workbook is designed to help you review what you have learned from reading your textbook. For this reason, the workbook is organized around learning objectives, just like the textbook and even your instructor's teaching material.

These learning objectives work as a built-in study guide. After completing the exercises for each learning objective in the workbook, ask yourself if you can DO what that learning objective describes.

If you can, move on to the next learning objective. If you cannot, just go back to the textbook, reread that learning objective, and try again.

We have provided procedure checklists close to the end of the workbook. The answers to the workbook exercises are in your instructor's teaching guide.

Happy Learning!

vi

Name: _____

1

Understanding Healthcare Settings

1. Discuss the structure of the healthcare system and describe ways it is changing

Multiple Choice
Circle the letter of the answer that best completes the statement or answers the question.

1. Another name for a long-term care facility (LTCF) is
   (A) Nursing home
   (B) Home health care
   (C) Assisted living facility
   (D) Adult daycare facility

2. Assisted living facilities are initially for
   (A) People who need around-the-clock intensive care
   (B) People who need some help with daily care
   (C) People who will die within six months
   (D) People who need to be in an acute care facility

3. Which of the following statements is true of adult daycare?
   (A) It takes place in the person's home.
   (B) It takes place in a facility during daytime working hours.
   (C) Most people in adult daycare are seriously ill or disabled.
   (D) Most serious surgeries are performed at adult daycare centers.

4. Care given by specialists to restore or improve function after an illness or injury is called
   (A) Acute care
   (B) Subacute care
   (C) Rehabilitation
   (D) Hospice care

5. Care given to people who have six months or less to live is called
   (A) Acute care
   (B) Subacute care
   (C) Rehabilitation
   (D) Hospice care

6. Home health aides
   (A) May clean or shop for groceries along with giving care
   (B) Have no contact with the client's family and/or friends
   (C) Do not have any supervision
   (D) Do not provide personal care

7. People who live in LTC facilities are usually called _____ because it is where they live for the duration of their stay.
   (A) Patients
   (B) Healthcare providers
   (C) Regulators
   (D) Residents

Matching
For each of the following terms, write the letter of the correct definition from the list below.

8. __A__ HMOs (health maintenance organizations)

9. __C__ Facilities

10. __D__ Managed care

11. __E__ Payers

12. __F__ PPOs (preferred provider organizations)

13. __B__ Providers

Name: _____

(A) Cost-control strategies that are replacing traditional insurance companies

(B) People or organizations that provide health care

(C) Places where care is delivered or administered

(D) A health plan that states that clients must use a particular doctor or group of doctors

(E) People or organizations paying for health-care services

(F) A network of providers that contract to provide health services to a group of people

2. Describe a typical long-term care facility

True or False
Mark each statement with either a "T" for true or an "F" for false.

1. __T__ Long-term care facilities may offer assisted living, subacute care, or specialized care.

2. __T__ Facilities that offer specialized care must have specially trained employees.

3. __F__ Nonprofit organizations cannot own long-term care facilities.

3. Describe residents who live in long-term care facilities

Multiple Choice

1. What is the most important thing for a nursing assistant to know about the residents in her care?
   (A) Whether or not residents have family close by
   (B) How long residents have been in the facility
   (C) That each resident is an individual with his or her own abilities and needs
   (D) When residents normally have visitors

2. More than half of residents in long-term care facilities (LTCF) are
   (A) Younger than 50 years old
   (B) Caucasian females
   (C) Black males
   (D) Developmentally disabled children

3. In general, residents who stay at a facility for more than six months
   (A) Need 24-hour care
   (B) Have caregivers available to them in the community
   (C) Are suffering from a terminal illness
   (D) Are likely to return to live in the community

4. Which of the following statements is true of dementia?
   (A) It is defined as the loss of an extremity, such as the loss of a leg.
   (B) It is not present in the majority of residents in long-term care facilities.
   (C) It has no effect on thinking, reasoning, and communicating.
   (D) It affects approximately 50 to 90 percent of residents in long-term care facilities.

Short Answer

5. Why do you think it is important to care for each resident as a whole person instead of treating only his or her disorders and disabilities?

   Its important to care for each resident as a whole person because they have many needs & they will go unmet if staff don't work at meeting them.

4. Explain policies and procedures

True or False

1. __T__ A policy is a course of action to be followed. For example, all healthcare information must remain confidential.

2. __T__ Facilities will have procedures for reporting information about residents.

3. __F__ It is all right to do tasks not listed in the job description if they are very simple.

4. __T__ Changes in residents should be reported to the nurse.

5. __F__ It is all right for nursing assistants to discuss their personal lives with residents.

6. __T__ Each step in a written procedure is important and must be strictly followed.

5. Describe the long-term care survey process

Multiple Choice

1. What is the purpose of surveys in long-term care facilities?
   (A) To count the number of residents
   (B) To refine the care-planning process
   (C) To study how well residents are cared for
   (D) To help the facility decide appropriate visiting hours

2. If a surveyor asks you a question you do not know the answer to, how should you respond?
   (A) Guess.
   (B) Offer information on another topic.
   (C) Tell the surveyor what you think he or she wants to hear.
   (D) Admit that you do not know, and find out the answer.

3. Which of the following statements is true of the Joint Commission?
   (A) Facilities are required to participate in the Joint Commission's surveys.
   (B) State surveys are the same as the Joint Commission's surveys.
   (C) The goal of the Joint Commission's survey process is to improve safety and quality of care.
   (D) The survey process does not check on performance relating to patient rights.

6. Explain Medicare and Medicaid

Short Answer

1. List two groups of people who qualify for Medicare.

   Two groups of people that qualify are people with permanet kidney failure and certain disabilities.

2. List the two parts of Medicare and what each helps pay for.

   Hospital Insurance helps pay for care in hospital, skilled nursing facility, care from home health agency. Medical Insurance helps pay for physician Services & various other medical services & equipment.

3. How is eligibility for Medicaid determined?

   It is determind by income and special circumstances.

7. Discuss the term "culture change" and describe Pioneer Network and The Eden Alternative

Short Answer

1. Define the term "culture change." List four examples of how you think elderly people can benefit from culture change.

_____

_____

_____

_____

_____

_____

_____

_____

_____

_____

_____

_____

_____

_____

_____

_____

_____

_____

_____

_____

_____

_____

_____

2

The Nursing Assistant and the Care Team

1. Identify the members of the care team and describe how the care team works together to provide care

Matching
Use each letter only once.

1. _____ Registered Nurse (RN)

2. _____ Licensed Practical Nurse (LPN) or Licensed Vocational Nurse (LVN)

3. _____ Nursing Assistant (NA or CNA)

4. _____ Medical Social Worker (MSW)

5. _____ Occupational Therapist (OT)

6. _____ Physical Therapist (PT)

7. _____ Physician or Doctor (MD)

8. _____ Registered Dietitian (RD)

9. _____ Speech-Language Pathologist (SLP)

10. _____ Activities Director

11. _____ Resident

(A) Performs delegated tasks, such as taking vital signs, providing personal care, and reporting observations to other care team members

(B) Diagnoses disease or disability and prescribes treatment

(C) Licensed professional who has completed one to two years of education and is able to administer medications and give treatments

(D) The care team revolves around this person and his or her condition, treatment, and progress.

(E) Administers therapy in the form of heat, cold, massage, ultrasound, electricity, and exercise to muscles, bones, and joints

(F) Teaches exercises to help the resident improve or overcome speech problems

(G) Trains residents to compensate for disabilities during ADLs and other activities

(H) Creates diets for residents with special needs

(I) Helps residents get support services, such as counseling

(J) Licensed professional who has completed two to four years of education and coordinates, manages, and provides skilled nursing care

(K) Helps residents socialize and stay active

2. Explain the nursing assistant's role

Word Search
Fill in the blanks in the list of NA duties below, then find the words in the word search.

Nursing assistants will:

1. Help with _____ care, such as bathing and hair care

2. Help with _____ needs

3. Help residents to move around
   _____

4. Encourage residents to eat and
   _____

5. Promote self-care and
   _____

Nursing assistants will NOT

6. Give _____ or insert or remove _____

Name: _____

```
i k n i r d m h t t y g k m
w f k n y k j y n o f l m h
h i s d q m x b b i n y z q
j z p e r s o n a l l r h e
f g f p b u s c a e s f a z
r v y e g u w g f t q j k r
v w s n o i t a c i d e m w
j n p d n d s o u n f l n o
e e t e s j p q x g s j h o
e x g n u d g t x h s w l l
d c n c v f k j l f z y w w
x d a e j j w s a u s r o w
r r i r c c g n a k h n q o
b z e n t l s m e i r y i y
```

3. Explain professionalism and list examples of professional behavior

Short Answer
Mark each of the following items with a "P" for professional behavior or a "U" for unprofessional behavior.

1. _____ Being on time for work

2. _____ Being neatly dressed and groomed

3. _____ Doing extra tasks not assigned to you

4. _____ Keeping resident information confidential

5. _____ Telling a resident about a bad date you had over the weekend

6. _____ Explaining what you are going to do before giving care

7. _____ Accepting a necklace from a resident as a birthday gift

8. _____ Following policies and procedures

9. _____ Asking questions when you are not sure of something

10. _____ Not washing your hands before giving care to residents

11. _____ Being a positive role model

Matching
Use each letter only once.

12. _____ Dependable

13. _____ Tolerant

14. _____ Conscientious

15. _____ Honest

16. _____ Unprejudiced

17. _____ Respectful

18. _____ Compassionate

19. _____ Empathetic

20. _____ Tactful

(A) Being caring, concerned, considerate, empathetic, and understanding

(B) Giving the same quality of care regardless of age, gender, sexual orientation, religion, race, ethnicity, or condition

(C) Being guided by a sense of right and wrong and having principles

(D) Valuing other people's individuality and treating others politely and kindly

(E) Speaking and acting without offending others

(F) Being truthful

(G) Getting to work on time and doing assigned tasks skillfully

(H) Putting aside your personal opinions and not judging others

(I) Entering into the feelings of others

4. Describe proper personal grooming habits

Multiple Choice

1. Why is good grooming so important?
   (A) It helps you get to work on time.
   (B) It helps you remember to document properly.
   (C) It affects how residents feel about the care you give.
   (D) Good grooming is not important.

2. How often should nursing assistants bathe or shower?
   (A) Once a week
   (B) Twice a week
   (C) Every other day
   (D) Daily

3. Nursing assistants should not use _____ before going to work.
   (A) Deodorant or antiperspirant
   (B) Mouthwash
   (C) Perfume or cologne
   (D) Shampoo

4. Hair should always be
   (A) Dirty
   (B) Tied back if it is long
   (C) Dyed
   (D) Cut short

5. Which of the following statements is true of clothing?
   (A) Clothing can be wrinkled.
   (B) Clothing should be very tight.
   (C) Clothing should be clean.
   (D) Clothing should be revealing.

6. What is one type of jewelry that can be worn to work?
   (A) Diamond ring
   (B) Watch
   (C) Bangle bracelets
   (D) Cuff links

7. Why should artificial nails or extenders not be worn to work?
   (A) They may not match the uniform.
   (B) Confused residents may want to eat them.
   (C) They make it more difficult to chart observations.
   (D) They harbor bacteria.

5. Explain the chain of command and scope of practice

Multiple Choice

1. Which of the following statements is true of the chain of command?
   (A) It describes the line of authority in a facility.
   (B) It is the same as the care team.
   (C) It details the survey process for each facility.
   (D) Nursing assistants are at the top of the chain of command.

2. Liability is a legal term that means
   (A) The line of authority in a facility
   (B) Ignoring a resident's call light
   (C) Someone can be held responsible for harming someone else
   (D) A task that a person was not trained for

3. Why is it important not to do tasks that are not assigned to you?
   (A) You may be assigned more work if you perform additional tasks.
   (B) You may put yourself or someone else in danger.
   (C) You may need to pay for additional training.
   (D) You may have to start arriving at work earlier.

4. What is one reason that other members of the care team will show great interest in the work that you do?
   (A) They may not trust you.
   (B) You will be working under the authority of others' licenses.
   (C) They may not have much respect for nursing assistants.
   (D) They can avoid having to pay you if you make a mistake.

Short Answer

5. Define "scope of practice."

_____

_____

_____

_____

_____

_____

_____

_____

6. List three tasks that are said to be outside the scope of practice of a nursing assistant.

_____

_____

_____

_____

_____

_____

_____

_____

_____

_____

_____

6. Define "care plan" and explain its purpose

True or False

1. _____ The purpose of the care plan is to give suggestions for care, which the nursing assistant can customize for each resident.

2. _____ Activities that are not listed on the care plan should not be performed.

3. _____ Care planning does not involve the resident's input or feelings.

4. _____ Sometimes even simple observations that nursing assistants make about residents are very important.

7. Describe the nursing process

Multiple Choice

1. The assessment step of the nursing process involves
   (A) Getting information about the resident and reviewing this information
   (B) Identifying health problems and resident needs
   (C) Setting goals and creating a care plan
   (D) Deciding if goals were met

2. The diagnosis step of the nursing process involves
   (A) Getting information about the resident and reviewing this information
   (B) Identifying health problems and resident needs
   (C) Deciding if goals were met
   (D) Putting the care plan into action

3. The planning step of the nursing process involves
   (A) Getting information about the resident and reviewing this information
   (B) Identifying health problems and resident needs
   (C) Putting the care plan into action
   (D) Setting goals and creating a care plan

4. The implementation step of the nursing process involves
   (A) Identifying health problems and resident needs
   (B) Putting the care plan into action
   (C) Setting goals and creating a care plan
   (D) Deciding if goals were met

5. The evaluation step of the nursing process involves
   (A) Identifying health problems and resident needs
   (B) Deciding if goals were met
   (C) Putting the care plan into action
   (D) Setting goals and creating a care plan

6. The goal of the nursing process is
   (A) To train the care team staff
   (B) To protect the facility from liability
   (C) To meet the resident's nursing needs
   (D) To keep resident information confidential

_____

_____

_____

_____

_____

_____

_____

8. Describe "The Five Rights of Delegation"

Fill in the Blank

Questions to ask before delegating a task include the following:

1. Is there a match between the resident's _____ and the NA's skills, _____, and experience?

2. What is the level of resident _____?

3. Can the nurse give appropriate direction and _____?

4. Is the nurse available to give _____, support, and help?

Questions to ask before accepting a task include the following:

5. Do I have all the _____ I need to do this job?

6. Do I have the necessary _____ for the task?

7. Do I have the needed supplies, _____ and other support?

8. Do I know how to reach my _____?

9. Demonstrate how to manage time and assignments

Short Answer

List five guidelines for managing time.

_____

_____

_____

Name: _____

3

Legal and Ethical Issues

1. Define the terms "law" and "ethics" and list examples of legal and ethical behavior

Short Answer

For each of the following examples, decide whether the issue is a legal issue or an ethical issue. Write "L" for "legal" or "E" for "ethical."

1. _____ Dorothy, a nursing assistant, makes fun of the way one of her residents speaks English when she is at home with her husband.

2. _____ Dennis, a nursing assistant, takes a necklace from a resident with dementia, whom he thinks will not notice, to give to his girlfriend.

3. _____ Lisa is ten minutes late coming in for work on Monday. Her supervisor does not notice and Lisa does not tell her.

4. _____ Paula is having trouble completing her procedures on time. She is afraid of losing her job, so she makes up a blood pressure reading on a resident's chart.

Read each of the following scenarios and answer the questions.

5. Sarah, a nursing assistant, is out shopping with her friends. One of them asks her if she likes her job, and she responds enthusiastically. She proceeds to relate to them that her resident, Mrs. Daly, has Alzheimer's disease and has to be reminded of her name several times a day, as she is apt to forget it.

Did Sarah behave in a legal and ethical manner? Why or why not?

_____

_____

_____

_____

_____

6. Caroyl, a nursing assistant, finishes her duties for the day and is about to leave. One of her residents, Mr. Leach, tells her how pleased he is with her work. He says that she is the first NA that has made him feel so comfortable and well taken care of. He gives her a little box of candy and says it is for all the hard work she has done. Caroyl initially refuses, but after he insists, she takes it from him, thanking him.

Did Caroyl behave in a legal and ethical manner? Why or why not?

_____

_____

_____

_____

_____

7. Mark, a nursing assistant, has been working at a facility for almost a year. One of his residents, Mrs. Hedman, has family visiting her from out-of-state. Mark meets her daughter, Susan, for the first time. During the course of conversation, Susan asks Mark to come have a drink with her so that they can talk about her mother's case in a more relaxed environment. Mark tells her that he can go out for a short while. They arrange to meet.

Did Mark behave in a legal and ethical manner? Why or why not?

_____

_____

_____

_____

_____

_____

_____

_____

_____

_____

2. Explain the Omnibus Budget Reconciliation Act (OBRA)

Multiple Choice

1. The Omnibus Budget Reconciliation Act (OBRA) sets minimum standards for
   (A) Facility cleanliness
   (B) Resident grooming
   (C) Nursing assistant training
   (D) Facility spending

2. According to OBRA, nursing assistants must complete at least ___ hours of training and must pass a competency evaluation before they can be employed.
   (A) 100
   (B) 250
   (C) 50
   (D) 75

3. The Minimum Data Set (MDS) is
   (A) Minimum staff requirements for each facility
   (B) Minimum services that nursing homes must provide
   (C) Minimum hours of training for NAs each year
   (D) Form for assessing residents and solving problems

4. An MDS must be completed for each resident
   (A) Within 14 days of admission and again each year and any time there is a change
   (B) Every six months
   (C) Never, unless a serious problem exists
   (D) Every two years

3. Explain residents' rights and discuss why they are important

Multiple Choice
Read each of the following scenarios. Decide which of the residents' rights is being violated in each, and circle the letter.

1. Mrs. Perkins is a visually impaired resident. She is very nearsighted and has misplaced her glasses many times. She gets upset during eye examinations, so the staff at her facility often allow her to go without glasses for a few weeks before having them replaced. Which of the residents' rights are violated in this case?
   (A) Services and activities to maintain a high level of wellness
   (B) The right to complain
   (C) The right to make independent choices
   (D) The right to privacy and confidentiality

2. Mr. Gallerano has a stomach ulcer that gives him minor pain. He has medication for it, but he says that it makes him nauseous and he does not want to take it. Lila, a nursing assistant, tells him that he may not have his dinner until he takes the medication. Which residents' right is Lila violating?
   (A) The right to be fully informed about rights and services
   (B) The right to participate in their own care
   (C) The right to security of possessions
   (D) The right to privacy and confidentiality

3. Ms. Mayes, a resident with severe arthritis, has a blue sweater that she loves to wear. The buttons are very tiny, and she cannot button them herself. Jim, a nursing assistant, tells her that she cannot wear the sweater today because it takes him too long to help her into it. Which residents' right has Jim violated?
   (A) The right to make independent choices
   (B) The right to participate in their own care
   (C) The right to be fully informed about rights and services
   (D) The right to privacy and confidentiality

4. Amy is a nursing assistant at Sweetwater Retirement Home. Every night when she goes home, she tells her family funny stories about the residents she is working with. Which residents' right is Amy violating?
   (A) The right to be fully informed about rights and services
   (B) The right to participate in their own care
   (C) The right to make independent choices
   (D) The right to privacy and confidentiality

5. Laura, a nursing assistant at Great Oak Nursing Home, is running behind with her work for the evening. She is helping Mr. Young, a resident with Alzheimer's, with his dinner. She is getting frustrated with him because he keeps taking the fork out of her hand and dropping it on the floor. Finally, she slaps his hand to get him to stop. Which residents' right has she violated?
   (A) The right to security of possessions
   (B) The right to complain
   (C) The right to dignity, respect, and freedom
   (D) The right to visits

6. Mrs. Hart is a resident with dementia at Longmeadow Retirement Home. She is usually unresponsive to her surroundings. James, a nursing assistant, notices a pretty bracelet on her dresser. He borrows it for his wife to wear to a formal dinner party, knowing that Mrs. Hart will not notice. Which residents' right has he violated?
   (A) The right to security of possessions
   (B) The right to complain
   (C) The right to make independent choices
   (D) The right to visits

7. Ms. Land, an elderly resident, gets into a loud argument with another resident during a card game. When her daughter comes to see her later that day, Anne, an NA, tells her that Ms. Land is in a bad mood and cannot see anyone. Which residents' right is she violating?
   (A) The right to security of possessions
   (B) Transfer and discharge rights
   (C) The right to make independent choices
   (D) The right to visits

8. During dinner, Pete, a nursing assistant, spills hot soup on a resident's arm. He tells her that she had better not tell anyone about it or he will be very angry at her. Which residents' right is he violating?
   (A) The right to security of possessions
   (B) Transfer and discharge rights
   (C) The right to visits
   (D) The right to complain

4. Discuss abuse and neglect and explain how to report abuse and neglect

Matching

1. _____ Abuse
2. _____ Active neglect
3. _____ Assault
4. _____ Battery
5. _____ Domestic violence
6. _____ Financial abuse
7. _____ Involuntary seclusion
8. _____ Negligence
9. _____ Passive neglect
10. _____ Physical abuse
11. _____ Psychological abuse
12. _____ Sexual abuse
13. _____ Sexual harassment
14. _____ Substance abuse
15. _____ Verbal abuse
16. _____ Workplace violence

(A) Actions or failure to act or provide proper care resulting in injury to a person

(B) The use of legal or illegal drugs, cigarettes, or alcohol in a way that harms oneself or others

(C) Any unwelcome sexual advance or behavior that creates an intimidating or hostile work environment

(D) Purposely harming a person physically, mentally, or emotionally by failing to give needed or correct care

Name: _____

(E) Confinement or separation from others without consent

(F) Abuse of caregivers or team members by residents or other team members

(G) Touching a person without his or her permission

(H) Threatening to touch a person without his or her permission

(I) Stealing, taking advantage of, or improperly using the money or other assets of another

(J) Forcing a person to perform or participate in sexual acts

(K) Oral or written words, pictures, or gestures that threaten, embarrass, or insult another person.

(L) Any behavior that causes the resident to feel threatened, fearful, intimidated, or humiliated

(M) Abuse by spouses, intimate partners, or family members

(N) Purposely causing physical, mental, or emotional pain or injury to someone

(O) Intentional or unintentional treatment that causes harm to a person's body

(P) Unintentionally harming a person physically, mentally, or emotionally by failing to give needed or correct care

Short Answer

17. Name five "suspicious" injuries that should be reported.

_____

_____

_____

_____

_____

_____

18. What are seven signs that could indicate abuse?

_____

_____

_____

_____

_____

_____

_____

19. What are seven signs that could indicate neglect?

_____

_____

_____

_____

_____

_____

_____

20. What are mandated reporters?

_____

_____

_____

_____

_____

_____

_____

21. If a resident wants to make a complaint of abuse, what must you do?

_____

_____

_____
_____
_____
_____
_____

5. List examples of behavior supporting and promoting residents' rights

Multiple Choice

1. When performing procedures on residents, you should
   (A) Try to distract them so they will not know what you are doing
   (B) Explain the procedure fully before performing it
   (C) Wait until they are sleeping before you start the procedure
   (D) Always notify the physician first

2. If a resident refuses to take a bath, you should
   (A) Offer her a prize if she will take the bath
   (B) Respect her wishes, but report it to the nurse
   (C) Tell her you will not answer the call light next time if she does not comply
   (D) Force her to take the bath

3. If your husband asks you to tell a story about a resident in your care, you should
   (A) Explain that you cannot talk or gossip about your resident
   (B) Tell him a story
   (C) Tell him a story, but only if he promises not to tell anyone else
   (D) Tell him something that you know that the resident would not mind you sharing

4. If you suspect your resident is being abused, you should
   (A) Open his mail and look through his belongings to find any clues
   (B) Call your closest friends and ask their advice
   (C) Report it to the nurse immediately
   (D) Check with his relatives first

6. Describe what happens when a complaint of abuse is made against a nursing assistant

Short Answer

What happens when a facility has determined that a nursing assistant abused a resident?

_____
_____
_____
_____
_____
_____
_____
_____
_____
_____
_____

7. Explain how disputes may be resolved and identify the ombudsman's role

Multiple Choice

1. One task of an ombudsman is to
   (A) Decide which special diet is right for a resident
   (B) Investigate and resolve resident complaints
   (C) Diagnose disease and prescribe medication
   (D) Take a resident's vital signs and report to the nurse

2. An ombudsman is assigned by law as the _____ advocate for residents.
   (A) Litigious
   (B) Liable
   (C) Lawyer
   (D) Legal

3. A Residents' Council meets to discuss issues related to the care facility. It is mostly made up of
   (A) Administrators
   (B) Directors of nursing
   (C) Residents
   (D) Nursing assistants

8. Explain HIPAA and list ways to protect residents' privacy

Multiple Choice

1. What is the purpose of HIPAA?
   (A) To monitor quality of care in facilities
   (B) To keep protected health information private and secure
   (C) To reduce incidents of abuse in facilities
   (D) To provide training for facility staff

2. What is included under protected health information (PHI)?
   (A) Patient's favorite food
   (B) Patient's favorite color
   (C) Patient's social security number and medical record number
   (D) Patient's library card number

3. What is the correct response if someone without a legal need to know asks for a resident's PHI?
   (A) Give them the information
   (B) Ask the resident if they may have the information
   (C) Ask them to send a written request for the information
   (D) Tell them that the information is confidential and cannot be given out

4. To protect residents' privacy, a nursing assistant should
   (A) Bring her family to the facility to meet residents
   (B) Discuss residents' progress with a co-worker in a restaurant
   (C) Use confidential rooms for reporting on residents
   (D) Let anyone calling the facility know the status of residents' conditions

9. Explain The Patient Self-Determination Act (PSDA) and discuss advance directives

Matching

1. _____ Advance directives

2. _____ Living will

3. _____ Durable power of attorney for health care

4. _____ Do-not-resuscitate (DNR) order

(A) A signed, dated, and witnessed paper that appoints someone else to make the medical decisions for a person in the event he or she becomes unable to do so.

(B) States the medical care a person wants, or does not want, in case he or she becomes unable to make those decisions him- or herself.

(C) Legal documents that allow people to choose what medical care they wish to have if they cannot make those decisions themselves.

(D) A legal document that tells medical professionals not to perform CPR (cardiopulmonary resuscitation).

4

Communication and Cultural Diversity

1. Define the term "communication"

Short Answer

1. List the three basic steps of communication.

    _____

    _____

    _____

2. Why is feedback an important part of communication?

    _____

    _____

    _____

    _____

3. With whom must nursing assistants be able to communicate?

    _____

    _____

    _____

    _____

Multiple Choice

4. Which three things are needed for communication to take place?
    (A) Signs, symbols, and drawings
    (B) Sender, receiver, and feedback
    (C) Supervisor, residents, and family members
    (D) Loud voice, ability to speak, resident's chart

5. The three-step process of communication occurs
    (A) Only once
    (B) Over and over
    (C) Only in formal meetings with the care team
    (D) In a different order every time

2. Explain verbal and nonverbal communication

Multiple Choice

1. Which of the following is an example of nonverbal communication?
    (A) Asking for a glass of water
    (B) Pointing to a glass of water
    (C) Screaming for a glass of water
    (D) Saying you do not like water

2. Types of verbal communication include:
    (A) Facial expressions
    (B) Nodding your head
    (C) Speaking
    (D) Shrugging your shoulders

3. Which of the following is an example of a confusing or conflicting message (saying one thing and meaning another)?
    (A) Mr. Carter smiles happily and tells you he is excited because his daughter is coming to visit.
    (B) Mrs. Sanchez looks like she is in pain. When you ask her about it, she tells you that her back has been bothering her.
    (C) Ms. Jones agrees with you when you say it is a nice day, but she looks angry.
    (D) Mr. Lee will not watch his favorite TV show. He says he is a little depressed.

4. In the previous question, how would you clarify the confusing or conflicting message?
   (A) Tell the person that you know they are not telling the truth.
   (B) Ignore the conflicting message and accept what the person has told you.
   (C) Ask the person to repeat what he or she has just said.
   (D) State what you have observed and ask if the observation is correct.

Short Answer

State whether each behavior below sends a positive message or a negative message to the receiver. Write "P" for "positive" and "N" for "negative."

5. _____ An impatient or angry tone

6. _____ Smiling

7. _____ Leaning forward in your chair

8. _____ Glancing repeatedly at your watch

9. _____ Sitting up straight

10. _____ Slouching

11. _____ Crossing your arms in front of your body

12. _____ Listening carefully

13. _____ Hugs and warm touches

14. _____ Rolling your eyes

3. Describe ways different cultures communicate

Matching
Use each letter only once.

1. _____ Positive responses to it include acceptance and knowledge

2. _____ Learned behaviors that are the tradition of a group of people and are passed on

3. _____ Prejudice

(A) Bias

(B) Cultural diversity

(C) Culture

Short Answer

4. What are four ways that people communicate nonverbally that are shaped by culture?

_____

_____

_____

_____

_____

5. What are some things that you can do to improve your awareness of your residents' cultures and needs?

_____

_____

_____

_____

6. Why do you think it is especially important in the United States to be accepting of cultural diversity?

_____

_____

_____

_____

_____

4. Identify barriers to communication

Crossword
Across

2. Your resident or the family may not understand _____ terms. Speak in simple, everyday words.

4. Avoid using _____ words that are unprofessional.

6. Be _____ with a resident who is difficult to understand.

8. Do not give medical _____ to the resident or family.

10. Keep in mind that _____ language is also part of your message, and be aware of it.

11. Make sure you speak clearly, especially if your resident is hard of _____.

Down

1. Ask _____ questions to get more information from the resident.

3. "Yes" or "no" answers bring the _____ to an end.

5. _____ are phrases used over and over again that do not really mean anything.

7. Do not offer your personal _____ or give advice to the resident or family.

9. Avoid asking _____ when your resident makes a statement.

5. List ways to make communication accurate and explain how to develop effective interpersonal relationships

Multiple Choice

1. One way to be a good listener is to
   (A) Finish a resident's sentences for him to show that you understand what he is saying
   (B) Pretend that you understand what a resident is saying even if you do not
   (C) Restate the message in your own words
   (D) Fill in any pauses to avoid awkwardness

2. Active listening involves
   (A) Focusing on the sender and giving feedback
   (B) Avoiding speaking to the resident if you cannot understand her
   (C) Finishing a resident's sentences for her if you know what he is going to say
   (D) Talking about personal problems you have been having at home

3. Mrs. Velasco is a new resident at Summerhill Retirement Home. Simon, a nursing assistant, is giving her a bath before bedtime. He notices that she seems to have difficulty speaking English and seems nervous. What can Simon do to make her more comfortable?
   (A) Give her advice about how to fit in better with American culture
   (B) Finish her sentences for her so that she will not have to speak
   (C) Use some words and phrases that he is familiar with in her language
   (D) Avoid speaking to her while giving care

4. When residents report symptoms or feelings, it is a good idea to
   (A) Interrupt the resident
   (B) Ignore the resident
   (C) Avoid speaking
   (D) Ask for more information

Name: _____

5. Which of the following statements reflects a way for nursing assistants to have good relationships with residents?
   (A) An NA should fold her arms in front of her while the resident is talking.
   (B) An NA should chat with other staff members if the resident she is assisting is unable to talk.
   (C) An NA should ignore a resident's request if she knows she cannot fulfill it.
   (D) An NA should be empathic and try to understand what residents are going through.

6. Mr. Vernon is an elderly resident who has terminal cancer. He is telling Katie, a nursing assistant, that he is very depressed about dying. He feels he has left many things unfinished. Hearing these things makes Katie uncomfortable. How should she respond?
   (A) Ignore what he is saying
   (B) Try to interest him in a brighter subject
   (C) Listen to the resident and ask questions when appropriate
   (D) Tell him she knows how he feels

7. During conversations with a resident, a nursing assistant should
   (A) Talk to other staff members
   (B) Use affectionate terms such as "dear" and "honey"
   (C) Call the resident by the name the resident prefers
   (D) Avoid using the resident's name

6. Explain the difference between facts and opinions

Fact or Opinion
For each statement, decide whether it is an example of a fact or an opinion. Write "F" for fact or "O" for opinion in the space provided.

1. _____ Mr. Ellington sounds angry.

2. _____ Mr. Wells did not speak to me when I was cleaning his room and was crying when I came in.

3. _____ Ms. Crainz has not been getting enough to eat.

4. _____ Ms. Porter did not drink any of her milk at dinnertime.

5. _____ I think Mr. Holling is lonely.

6. _____ Mr. Larking's pulse was elevated last night after dinner, but it was back to normal this morning.

7. _____ Mr. Perry and his new roommate are not getting along.

8. _____ Mr. Peterson became agitated while preparing for his bath and refused to wash his hair.

9. _____ Mrs. Myers needs assistance to stand up.

10. _____ Mrs. Myers looks like she is in a lot of pain.

11. _____ Mr. Ford drinks more coffee than is good for him.

12. _____ Mr. Ford drinks three cups of coffee every morning.

Scenario

Karen is a nursing assistant at Greenhollow Nursing Home. She has just finished assisting Ms. Lynn, a resident with Alzheimer's disease, with her dinner. She is discussing the events of the meal with her supervisor. Read Karen's statement. Indicate which parts of her report are statements of fact, and which are statements of opinion.

"Ms. Lynn was grouchy at dinner today. She said that she did not like the peas and that the milk she has been drinking makes her nauseous. Actually, she did look a little queasy. She liked the meat loaf but she did not like the peas or the milk. She ate all of the meat, but none of the peas. She only had two sips of milk. During dessert, she got a little depressed. She stopped talking to me and the other residents and only had one bite of her brownie."

Name: _____

_____
_____
_____
_____
_____
_____
_____
_____
_____
_____
_____
_____
_____
_____
_____
_____

Labeling
Looking at the diagram, list examples of observations using each sense.

Smell: _____
_____
_____
_____

Sight: _____
_____
_____
_____

Hearing: _____
_____
_____

Touch: _____
_____
_____
_____

7. Explain objective and subjective information and describe how to observe and report accurately

Short Answer
For each of the following, decide whether it is an objective observation (you can see, hear, smell, or touch it) or subjective observation (the resident must tell you about it). Write "O" for objective and "S" for subjective.

1. _____ Skin rash
2. _____ Crying
3. _____ Rapid pulse
4. _____ Headache
5. _____ Nausea
6. _____ Vomiting
7. _____ Swelling
8. _____ Cloudy urine
9. _____ Wheezing
10. _____ Feeling sad

8. Explain how to communicate to other team members

Multiple Choice

1. When giving information to other members of the care team about a resident, a nursing assistant should
   (A) Discuss it in the hallway around other residents
   (B) Make a diagnosis of the resident's condition
   (C) Share information with anyone who asks about the resident's condition
   (D) Make sure that she respects the resident's right to privacy

2. The health professional who should give a resident's family and friends information about any new diagnoses is
   (A) A doctor
   (B) A nursing assistant
   (C) An activities director
   (D) A music therapist

9. Describe basic medical terminology and abbreviations

Matching
For each of the following abbreviations, write the letter of the correct term from the list below.

1. _____ ac
2. _____ amb
3. _____ BM
4. _____ C
5. _____ c/o
6. _____ CPR
7. _____ F
8. _____ ft
9. _____ GI
10. _____ hs
11. _____ I&O
12. _____ NPO
13. _____ OOB
14. _____ pc
15. _____ PRN
16. _____ R
17. _____ ROM
18. _____ SOB
19. _____ VS
20. _____ w/c

(A) Fahrenheit degree

(B) hours sleep

(C) after meals

(D) nothing by mouth

(E) bowel movement

(F) cardiopulmonary resuscitation

(G) complains of

(H) range of motion

(I) respirations

(J) vital signs

(K) shortness of breath

(L) before meals

(M) foot

(N) wheelchair

(O) as necessary

(P) intake and output

(Q) Celsius degree

(R) out of bed

(S) gastrointestinal

(T) ambulate

10. Explain how to give and receive an accurate report of a resident's status

Multiple Choice

1. Which of the following is true of oral reports?
   (A) Nursing assistants should use mostly facts when making oral reports.
   (B) Nursing assistants should use mostly opinions when making oral reports.
   (C) Nursing assistants should make oral reports directly to residents' families and friends.
   (D) Nursing assistants do not need to make oral reports; they only need to make written reports.

2. Report information will be shared with
   (A) Residents' friends and families
   (B) Other residents on the same floor
   (C) The nursing assistant's family
   (D) Members of the care team

3. Which of the following should be reported to the nurse immediately?
   (A) Trouble sleeping
   (B) Falls
   (C) Visits from family
   (D) Requests for toileting assistance

4. What is the best way to remember important details for an oral report?
   (A) Rely on your memory
   (B) Repeat the information to a friend or another resident
   (C) Write notes and use them for your report
   (D) Tell another nursing assistant to remind you

11. Explain documentation and describe related terms and forms

Multiple Choice

1. The large amount of time that a nursing assistant spends with residents will allow her to
   (A) Diagnose resident illnesses
   (B) Determine treatment
   (C) Notice things about residents that other care team members may not notice
   (D) Give medications to residents

2. Which of the following is true of a resident's medical chart?
   (A) A medical chart is the legal record of a resident's care.
   (B) All care does not need to be documented.
   (C) Documentation can be put off until the nursing assistant has time to do it.
   (D) Medical charts only contain the resident's name, address, and date of birth.

3. When should notes be written?
   (A) Before care is given
   (B) Immediately after care is given
   (C) At the end of the day
   (D) Whenever there is time

4. The Minimum Data Set (MDS) manual
   (A) Shows how residents should be transferred
   (B) Describes the line of authority in the facility
   (C) Helps the nurse complete accurate assessments
   (D) Gives procedures for reporting toxic spills

Short Answer

Convert the following regular times to military time.

5. 2:10 p.m. _____

6. 4:30 a.m. _____

7. 10:00 a.m. _____

8. 8:25 p.m. _____

Convert the following military times to regular time.

9. 0600 _____

10. 2320 _____

11. 1927 _____

12. 1800 _____

12. Describe incident reporting and recording

Multiple Choice

1. An incident is
   (A) An accident or unexpected event in the course of care
   (B) Any interaction between residents and staff
   (C) A normal part of facility routine
   (D) Any event in a resident's day

2. Which of the following would be considered an incident?
   (A) A resident complains of a headache.
   (B) A resident on a restricted-sodium diet receives and eats a regular, non-restricted meal.
   (C) A resident wants to watch TV in the common living area
   (D) A resident needs to be transferred from his bed to a chair.

3. Incidents should be reported to
   (A) The resident's family
   (B) The charge nurse
   (C) All staff on duty at the time of the incident
   (D) The doctor on call

True or False

4. _____ Documentation of incidents helps protect the resident, the employer, and individual staff members.

5. _____ The information in an incident report is confidential.

6. _____ If you do not actually see an incident but arrive after it has already occurred, you should document what you think happened.

7. ____ The documentation of an incident should include the name of the person responsible for the incident.

8. ____ Incident reports should be factual.

9. ____ It is inappropriate to include suggestions for improvement in an incident report.

10. ____ Do not report an incident that makes you feel uncomfortable unless you think it might be a direct threat to you.

11. ____ If you receive an injury on the job, you should file an incident report.

13. Demonstrate effective communication on the telephone

Scenarios
Read the following telephone conversations and think about how the nursing assistant could have better presented herself on the phone.

Example #1 Making a call from a facility

Hi, who's this?

Could you get Ms. Crier on the phone, please? I need to talk to her.

She's not there? Do you know where she is? I really have to talk to her right now. My resident asked me to call her to see if she can come visit today. She's really lonely and needs a visitor.

Okay, well tell her Ella called and have her call me back. Ella Ferguson. The number? I don't remember what it is. Just look up Whispering Pines Nursing Facility.

I don't know how much longer I'll be here, but have her call me as soon as possible. Bye.

1. What did the nursing assistant do wrong in this phone conversation?

_____

_____

_____

_____

_____

Example #2 Answering a call at a facility

Hello? Who? Julie Lee? No, she can't come to the phone right now. She's on her break outside and is smoking a cigarette. Who's calling?

And your number?

Can I tell her what this is about?

Okay. I'll give her the message. Goodbye.

2. What did the nursing assistant do wrong in this phone conversation?

_____

_____

_____

_____

_____

_____

_____

_____

_____

14. Understand guidelines for basic office machines and computers

Matching
For each of the following definitions, write the letter of the correct term from the list below.

1. ____ A machine that makes paper copies of documents and other images quickly

2. ____ A machine that performs mathematical calculations

3. _____ A system for sending and receiving messages electronically over a computer system or network

4. _____ A machine that transfers copies of documents over a telephone network

5. _____ Electronic devices that process and store information

6. _____ A worldwide communications system that links a network of computers

(A) Calculator

(B) Computers

(C) E-mail

(D) Fax machine

(E) Internet

(F) Photocopier or copier

15. Explain the resident call system

Multiple Choice

1. How do residents signal staff that they need assistance?
   (A) By calling out their names as they see them
   (B) By calling the nurses' station on the phone
   (C) By using a signal light or call light
   (D) By calling family members on the telephone

2. When is it acceptable to ignore a call light?
   (A) When you have just left a resident's room
   (B) When you are very busy
   (C) When the resident signaling is not assigned to you
   (D) Never

3. Call lights should be placed
   (A) Near the door of the resident's room
   (B) In a common area of the floor
   (C) Within reach of the resident
   (D) In any location that is convenient

16. List guidelines for communicating with residents with special needs

Fill in the Blank

Guidelines for Hearing-Impaired Residents

1. Make sure hearing-impaired residents are wearing their

   _____

   and that they are working properly.

2. Hearing aids should be cleaned

   _____.

3. Reduce or remove

   _____,

   such as TVs or radios.

4. Do not approach hearing-impaired residents from _____.

5. Keep your hands away from your

   _____

   when talking with hearing-impaired residents.

6. Use short

   _____ and

   simple _____.

7. Use _____
   cards as needed.

Fill in the Blank

Guidelines for Visually Impaired Residents

8. Do not _____
   the resident before identifying yourself.

9. Always tell the resident what you are doing while caring for him. Give specific

   _____,

   such as, "On your right" or, "In front of you."

10. Make sure there is proper

    _____

    in the room. Face the resident when you are speaking.

11. _____

    the resident to new areas. Describe the things you see around you.

12. Use the face of an imaginary

_____

to describe position of objects in front of the resident.

13. Do not _____ furniture or personal items without the resident's knowledge and permission.

14. Leave the door completely

_____ or

completely

_____ .

Matching

Guidelines for CVA

15. _____ Occurs when blood supply is cut off from the brain

16. _____ Weakness on one side of the body

17. _____ Paralysis on one side of the body

18. _____ Inability to speak or speak clearly

19. _____ Inability to understand spoken or written words

20. _____ Laughing or crying without reason

21. _____ Difficulty swallowing

(A) Receptive aphasia

(B) Emotional lability

(C) Hemiplegia

(D) Cerebrovascular accident

(E) Dysphagia

(F) Hemiparesis

(G) Expressive aphasia

Fill in the Blank

Guidelines for CVA

22. Keep questions and directions

_____ .

23. Ask questions that can be answered with a

_____ or

_____

24. Refer to the side of the resident's body with weakness or paralysis as the

_____ or

_____ side.

25. Keep _____ within reach of resident.

26. Use pictures, gestures, and

_____

boards to aid communication.

True or False

Guidelines for Combative and/or Angry Residents

27. _____ Combative behavior can be verbal as well as physical.

28. _____ Combative behavior usually occurs in reaction to a specific person.

29. _____ If combative behavior does not upset anyone, it does not need to be documented.

30. _____ It is never acceptable to hit a resident under any circumstances.

31. _____ Presenting logical arguments is a good way to counter combative behavior.

32. _____ Anger may be expressed through violent, aggressive behavior, or by withdrawal or sulking.

33. _____ Using silence may allow a resident to express why she is angry.

34. _____ Assertive behavior includes expressing thoughts, feelings, and beliefs in a direct and honest way.

True or False

Guidelines for Inappropriate Behavior

35. _____ Inappropriate behavior includes comments as well as physical actions.

36. _____ Illness, dementia, or medication may cause inappropriate behavior.

37. _____ You should try to distract the resident from behaving inappropriately.

38. _____ If you think that the resident's behavior is harmless, you do not need to report it.

39. _____ Hitting a resident for any reason is considered abuse.

5

Preventing Infection

1. Define "infection control" and related terms

Matching
Use each letter only once.

1. _____ Measures practiced in healthcare facilities to prevent and control the spread of disease

2. _____ A harmful microorganism

3. _____ Infections that patients acquire within healthcare settings that result from treatment for other conditions

4. _____ Tiny living thing that cannot be seen without a microscope

5. _____ The state of being free of all microorganisms, not just pathogens

6. _____ The process of removing pathogens, or the state of being free of pathogens

7. _____ An infection that is in the bloodstream and is spread throughout the body

8. _____ In healthcare, objects that have not been contaminated with pathogens

9. _____ Occurs when pathogens invade the body and multiply

10. _____ An infection that is confined to a specific location in the body

11. _____ In healthcare, objects that have been contaminated with pathogens

(A) Clean

(B) Dirty

(C) Healthcare-associated infection

(D) Infection

(E) Infection control

(F) Localized infection

(G) Medical asepsis

(H) Microorganism/microbe

(I) Pathogen

(J) Surgical asepsis

(K) Systemic infection

2. Describe the chain of infection

Word Search
Fill in the blanks in the description of the chain of infection below. Then find your answers in the word search.

1. A(n) _____ is a pathogen or microorganism that causes disease.

2. A(n) _____ is a place where a pathogen lives and grows.

3. An opening on an infected person that lets pathogens leave is a(n) _____.

4. Pathogens travel from one person to another through a mode of _____.

5. The _____ is an opening on an infected person that lets pathogens enter.

6. A(n) _____ host is an uninfected person who could get sick.

Name: _____

```
p m y o k y e f p s j z w u
e o b m w j a q o i j v b g
l s r d l e a h r e s b g g
b a c t o b k q t d b n h r
i j b o a b o i a u u m i j
t f v l n l v z l g k o p v
p r s e d j o o o u v k v g
e t c g z q m f f r y g g r
c a u s a t i v e a g e n t
s m k q e d k s x n h u g m
u p z c t g e h i q t z a c
s b m p n r n c t v w r r j
n o i s s i m s n a r t y d
o v n a b c p l f n u u u m
```

3. Explain why the elderly are at a higher risk for infection and identify symptoms of an infection

True or False

1. _____ The elderly have a higher risk for infection than younger people.

2. _____ It is normal for a person's immune system to grow weaker as he or she ages.

3. _____ Blood circulation is increased as a person ages.

4. _____ Limited mobility increases the risk of pressure sores among the elderly.

5. _____ Nutrition and fluid intake play no part in helping prevent infection.

6. _____ The elderly are less likely than younger people to have healthcare-associated infections.

7. _____ Infections are less dangerous in the elderly than in younger people.

8. _____ Nursing assistants play an important role in protecting elderly residents from infections.

9. _____ Redness and swelling are common symptoms of a systemic infection.

10. _____ Fever, chills, and mental confusion are symptoms of systemic infection.

4. Describe the Centers for Disease Control and Prevention (CDC) and explain Standard Precautions

True or False

1. _____ Standard Precautions means treating all blood, body fluids, non-intact skin, and mucous membranes as if they were infected with an infectious disease.

2. _____ Standard Precautions relate to all body fluids except saliva.

3. _____ You can usually tell if someone is infectious by looking at him.

4. _____ The Centers for Disease Control and Prevention is a government agency that issues information to protect the health of individuals and communities.

5. _____ You should wash your hands before putting on gloves.

6. _____ Syringes should be re-capped after use.

7. _____ Giving mouth care will require you to wear gloves.

8. _____ It is a good idea to wear a mask and protective goggles if you are emptying a bedpan.

9. _____ When cleaning a urinal, you do not need to wear gloves.

Multiple Choice

10. Standard Precautions should be practiced
    (A) Only on people who look like they have a bloodborne disease
    (B) On every single person in your care
    (C) Only on people who request that you follow them
    (D) Only on people who have tuberculosis

11. Standard Precautions include the following measures
    (A) Using your used or soiled gloves to gather clean equipment
    (B) Wearing gloves if there is a possibility you will come into contact with blood, body fluids, mucous membranes, or broken skin

(C) Touching body fluids with your bare hands

(D) Putting caps on used needles

12. Which of the following is true of transmission-based, or isolation, precautions?
    (A) You do not need to practice Standard Precautions if you practice Transmission-Based Precautions.
    (B) They are exactly the same as Standard Precautions.
    (C) They are practiced in addition to Standard Precautions.
    (D) They are never practiced at the same time that Standard Precautions are used.

5. Explain the term "hand hygiene" and identify when to wash hands

Multiple Choice

1. You will come into contact with microorganisms
   (A) Only in public areas of the facility
   (B) Only during direct contact with residents
   (C) Only during personal care procedures
   (D) Every time you touch something

2. The CDC defines hand hygiene as
   (A) Handwashing with soap and water and using alcohol-based hand rubs
   (B) Using only alcohol-based hand rubs
   (C) Rinsing hands with water
   (D) Not washing hands more than once per day

3. Alcohol-based hand rubs are used
   (A) With water for maximum effectiveness
   (B) When facilities have run out of antimicrobial soap
   (C) To prevent dry, cracked skin
   (D) In addition to washing with soap and water

4. Why is it a bad idea to wear artificial nails to work?
   (A) Residents may not like them.
   (B) They may be lost.
   (C) They harbor bacteria and increase risk of contamination.
   (D) They may be damaged by frequent handwashing.

5. How long should you use friction when lathering and washing your hands?
   (A) 2 minutes
   (B) 5 seconds
   (C) 18 seconds
   (D) 20 seconds

6. Discuss the use of personal protective equipment (PPE) in facilities

Short Answer
Mark an "X" next to the tasks that require you to wear gloves.

1. _____ Handling body fluids
2. _____ Potentially touching blood
3. _____ Brushing a resident's hair
4. _____ Answering the telephone
5. _____ Performing or assisting with perineal care
6. _____ Washing vegetables
7. _____ Putting clean sheets on an unoccupied bed
8. _____ Performing or assisting with mouth care
9. _____ Shaving a resident

Word Search
Complete each of the following sentences and find your answers in the word search.

10. A _____ should be worn when caring for residents with respiratory illnesses.

11. _____ provide protection for your eyes.

12. If there is a chance you could come into contact with _____ membranes or open wounds, you should wear _____.

13. A mask, gloves, goggles, and

    _____

    are all examples of PPE.

Name: _____

```
q y v f q n m h q i e f c s
g l o v e s z u s y w z u v
b o b r u h s a e t i o l p
k w g b u u r p p t c g q a
u d f g q w k j m u d m m t
o s l x l n w k m e s t m z
y c m c l e n y q i r r k p
d x p t t v s w j q i h g p
o w q t c a u s o i k s s e
o a q k k x y k o g h n r d
l o s w q b q p c z e j w a
b a q c c c j b c p i d k l
m a n y w w y f s j o e o u
k i f z f l u i d s v g c l
```

Scenarios

After Zoe washes her hands, she will put on her PPE. She is going into an area in which she needs to use Transmission-Based Precautions, so she will wear a gown, a mask, and goggles in addition to her gloves. Read the steps she takes and write down anything she does incorrectly.

14. First Zoe puts on her gown. She holds it out in front of her and shakes it open. She slips her arms into the sleeves and then ties the neck ties in a secure knot so that it will not come untied while she is working. She reaches behind her and, making sure all of her clothing is covered, ties the back ties.

_____

_____

_____

_____

_____

_____

_____

_____

_____

15. Zoe then puts on her mask. Being careful not to touch the mask where it touches her face, she ties the bottom strings first and then the top strings. She then puts on her goggles, making sure they fit snugly over her glasses.

_____

_____

_____

_____

_____

_____

_____

_____

_____

16. Zoe is right-handed, so she will put on her right glove first. She then uses her gloved hand to put on her other glove. She holds her hands out in front of her to smooth out the folds in the gloves. She looks closely at the gloves for tears or holes. She sees an area that is discolored but it is very small, so she decides to wear the glove anyway. She pulls the sleeves of her gown over the cuffs of the gloves and is ready to get to work.

_____

_____

_____

_____

_____

_____

_____

_____

_____

7. List guidelines for handling equipment and linen

Matching
Use each word only once.

1. ____ A measure that destroys all microorganisms, including pathogens

2. ____ A process that kills pathogens, but not all microorganisms

3. ____ Only to be used once and then discarded

(A) Disinfection

(B) Disposable

(C) Sterilization

Fill in the Blank

4. Handle equipment to avoid skin or
_____
membrane contact.

5. Avoid _____
of your clothing. Hold linen and clothing
_____
from your uniform.

6. Prevent transfer of disease to other residents and areas by not _____
linen or clothes; fold or roll linen so that the dirtiest area is _____.

7. _____ and reprocess reusable equipment properly before using again. _____ of single-use, or disposable, equipment properly.

8. Bag soiled linen at the point of
_____.

9. Clean and disinfect all frequently touched
_____,
such as call lights.

10. Place _____
linen in leak-proof bags.

8. Explain how to handle spills

True or False

1. ____ You do not need to wear gloves to clean up a small spill.

2. ____ Place a disinfectant directly on the spilled fluid before absorbing and removing the fluid.

3. ____ It is OK to use your hands to pick up large pieces of broken glass and use a broom and dustpan for smaller pieces.

4. ____ Waste containing blood or body fluids should be disposed of in the trash can in the cafeteria.

5. ____ An absorbing powder may be used to absorb the spill before removing it.

9. Explain Transmission-Based Precautions

Matching
Match each definition or phrase below to the type of precaution described. Use an "A" for Airborne Precautions, a "C" for Contact Precautions, and a "D" for Droplet Precautions. Each letter may be used more than once.

1. ____ Transmission can occur with skin-to-skin contact during transfers or bathing.

2. ____ Used when there is a risk of transmitting or contracting a microorganism from touching an infected object or person

3. ____ Used to guard against tuberculosis and measles

4. ____ Covering your nose and mouth with a tissue when you sneeze or cough, and washing your hands immediately after sneezing on them, are parts of these precautions.

5. ____ Helps prevent the spread of lice and bacterial conjunctivitis

6. ____ Used when the microorganisms do not stay suspended in the air and travel only short distances (not more than three feet)

7. ____ Microorganisms can be created by coughing, sneezing, talking, laughing, or suctioning.

8. ____ Helps prevent the spread of illnesses transmitted through the air

9. ____ Helps protects against transmission of mumps

10. ____ May require the use of a special mask, such as an N-95 or HEPA mask

Multiple Choice

11. Transmission-Based Precautions are used
    (A) Every day on the job
    (B) In addition to Standard Precautions
    (C) Instead of Standard Precautions
    (D) When treating all residents with terminal illnesses

12. Dedicated equipment refers to
    (A) Equipment that is used by multiple residents
    (B) Equipment donated to one resident by another resident and/or his family
    (C) Equipment that is disposable
    (D) Equipment that is only used by one resident

13. Which of the following is true of wearing PPE while caring for residents in isolation?
    (A) Nursing assistants will have to decide for themselves which PPE they must wear while caring for residents in isolation.
    (B) Nursing assistants should remove PPE before exiting a resident's room.
    (C) Nursing assistants will always wear the same PPE while caring for all residents in isolation.
    (D) Nursing assistants should remove PPE after exiting a resident's room.

14. When a resident is in isolation,
    (A) He or she should be avoided until the time in isolation is completed.
    (B) Nursing assistants must perform all tasks requested of them, even if they are outside the scope of practice.
    (C) He or she has the same basic human needs.
    (D) Nursing assistants should leave uneaten food in the resident's room for 24 hours to see if he or she will eat it.

10. Define "bloodborne pathogens" and describe two major bloodborne diseases

Multiple Choice

1. Bloodborne diseases can be transmitted by
   (A) Infected blood entering your bloodstream
   (B) Hugging a person with a bloodborne disease
   (C) Being in the same room as a person with a bloodborne disease
   (D) Talking to a person with a bloodborne disease

2. In health care, the most common way to get a bloodborne disease is by
   (A) Contact with infected blood or certain body fluids
   (B) Hugging a resident with a bloodborne disease
   (C) Being in the same room as a resident with a bloodborne disease
   (D) Sexual contact with residents

3. How does the human immunodeficiency virus (HIV) affect the body?
   (A) It cuts off blood supply to the brain.
   (B) It causes hearing impairment by damaging the inner ear.
   (C) It causes diabetes in otherwise healthy people.
   (D) It weakens the immune system so that the body cannot fight infection.

4. Which of the following is true of hepatitis B (HBV)?
   (A) HBV is caused by fecal-oral contamination.
   (B) There is no vaccine for HBV.
   (C) HBV is caused by jaundice.
   (D) HBV can be transmitted through blood or needles that are contaminated with the virus.

5. Your employer must offer a free vaccine to protect you from
   (A) HIV/AIDS
   (B) Hepatitis B
   (C) Hepatitis E
   (D) All bloodborne diseases

11. Explain OSHA's Bloodborne Pathogen Standard

Multiple Choice

1. The Occupational Safety and Health Administration (OSHA) is a federal government agency that protects workers from
    (A) Unfair employment practices
    (B) Lawsuits
    (C) Workplace violence
    (D) Hazards on the job

2. The Bloodborne Pathogens Standard is a law that requires that
    (A) Healthcare employers must have a written exposure control plan designed to eliminate or reduce employee exposure to infectious material
    (B) Healthcare employers must only accept residents who are healthy upon admission
    (C) Healthcare employers must charge employees $15 for hepatitis B vaccinations
    (D) Healthcare employers must disclose information about residents' diagnoses to the public

3. Which of the following does OSHA consider significant exposures?
    (A) Needle sticks
    (B) Clean utility rooms
    (C) PPE
    (D) Hand hygiene

4. According to OSHA, employers must give all employees, residents, and visitors _____ to use when needed.
    (A) Syringes
    (B) Manual Data Set (MDS) assessments
    (C) PPE
    (D) Medical charts

5. Why is it important for employees to report any potential exposures immediately?
    (A) So that the employees can be terminated to avoid infecting others
    (B) To cover up any negligence on the part of the facility
    (C) To protect the employees' health and the health of others
    (D) So that employees can warn the residents of a possible epidemic

12. Define "tuberculosis" and list infection control guidelines

Multiple Choice

1. Tuberculosis may be transmitted
    (A) By coughing
    (B) By dancing
    (C) By wearing gloves
    (D) Through a protective mask

2. Tuberculosis is
    (A) A bloodborne disease
    (B) An airborne disease
    (C) A non-infectious disease
    (D) An untreatable disease

3. Someone with latent TB (TB infection)
    (A) Shows symptoms
    (B) Falls into a coma almost immediately
    (C) Cannot infect others
    (D) Can infect others

4. A person with active TB
    (A) Can infect others
    (B) Does not show symptoms
    (C) Cannot eat whole foods
    (D) Cannot walk on his or her own

5. TB disease is more likely to develop in people
    (A) Who live near the mountains
    (B) Whose relatives had it when they were kids
    (C) Whose immune systems are weakened
    (D) Who work alone

6. One major factor in the spread of TB is
    (A) Following isolation precautions if indicated in the care plan
    (B) Following Standard Precautions
    (C) Wearing a gown and mask during resident care
    (D) Failure to take all the medication prescribed

13. Define the terms "MRSA," "VRE," and "C. Difficile"

True or False

1. _____ MRSA is almost always spread by direct physical contact.

2. _____ Once VRE is established, it is relatively easy to get rid of it.

3. _____ MRSA can be spread through indirect contact by touching contaminated objects.

4. _____ Handwashing will not help control the spread of MRSA.

5. _____ VRE causes life-threatening infections in people with compromised immune systems.

6. _____ You can help prevent the spread of VRE by washing your hands often.

7. _____ Proper handwashing and handling of contaminated wastes can help prevent *Clostridium difficile*.

8. _____ Increasing the use of antibiotics helps lower the risk of developing *C. difficile* diarrhea.

14. List employer and employee responsibilities for infection control

Short Answer
Read the following and mark "er" for employer or "ee" for employee to show who is responsible for infection control.

1. _____ Immediately report any exposure you have to infection.

2. _____ Provide personal protective equipment for use and train how to properly use it.

3. _____ Follow all facility policies and procedures.

4. _____ Take advantage of the free hepatitis B vaccination.

5. _____ Provide continuing in-service education on infection control.

6. _____ Establish infection control procedures and an exposure control plan.

7. _____ Follow resident care plans and assignments.

8. _____ Participate in annual education programs covering infection control.

9. _____ Have written procedures to follow should an exposure occur.

6

Safety and Body Mechanics

1. Identify the persons at greatest risk for accidents and describe accident prevention guidelines

Short Answer

1. Why do the elderly have more safety concerns than younger people?

_____

_____

_____

_____

2. What is the key to safety in facilities?

_____

_____

_____

_____

_____

Word Search
Fill in the blanks below on guarding against falls, and then find your answers in the word search.

3. Keep all walking areas free of

_____ ,

trash, throw rugs, and cords.

4. Leave

_____

in the same place as you found it.

5. Answer _____
   right away.

6. Return beds to their

_____

position after giving care.

7. Keep frequently-used personal items
   _____ to residents.

8. Lock _____
   before helping residents into or out of them.

9. Make sure residents'

_____ are tied
   and that they are wearing non-slip shoes.

10. Immediately clean up

_____

on the floor.

11. Offer help with

_____

regularly and respond to requests for help
immediately.

12. Lock _____
    wheels before helping a resident into and
    out of bed or when giving care.

j	b	w	i	v	c	v	h	h	t	c	r	c	f
i	x	b	h	h	r	a	h	s	s	f	e	a	a
s	p	e	f	e	s	m	e	y	u	b	t	l	j
z	g	d	d	o	e	w	l	r	g	j	t	l	n
s	x	c	h	u	o	l	n	w	v	m	u	l	n
c	z	s	t	l	g	i	c	v	f	j	l	i	i
t	o	d	y	p	t	n	c	h	i	f	c	g	q
r	v	u	z	u	x	p	i	l	a	h	f	h	a
s	n	x	r	b	o	o	p	t	o	i	y	t	m
e	u	e	s	p	i	l	l	s	e	s	r	s	p
s	e	c	a	l	e	o	h	s	f	l	e	s	i
j	x	d	b	a	o	u	p	y	h	b	i	p	a
g	z	t	y	w	m	p	s	n	q	t	o	o	g
x	a	w	m	c	b	j	n	s	f	t	t	v	t

Multiple Choice

Burns/Scalds

13. Those at greatest risk for burns are
    (A) Administrators
    (B) Facility staff and their friends
    (C) Small children, older adults, and those with loss of sensation
    (D) All people are at equal risk for burns.

14. Scalds are burns caused by
    (A) Hot liquids
    (B) Stoves or other appliances
    (C) Cooking
    (D) Heating devices

15. How long does it take for a serious burn to occur with a liquid at a temperature of 140 °F?
    (A) 5 seconds or less
    (B) 10 seconds or more
    (C) 30 seconds or more
    (D) 20 seconds or more

16. How should you check the temperature of hot water?
    (A) Let the resident taste it and let you know
    (B) Guess based on how long it has been heating
    (C) With a water thermometer
    (D) With a stethoscope

17. What should you do if an appliance has a frayed cord or looks unsafe?
    (A) Report it immediately and stop using it.
    (B) Report it immediately but continue to use it until it is replaced.
    (C) Repair it yourself.
    (D) Continue to use it; it has probably already been reported.

18. When serving hot liquids to residents, you should
    (A) Pour hot drinks as close as possible to residents.
    (B) Pour hot drinks away from residents.
    (C) Keep hot liquids close to the edges of tables.
    (D) Ask the resident to stand up before serving the hot drink.

Short Answer

Resident Identification

19. What can happen if you do not identify a resident before mealtimes or giving care?

    _____

    _____

    _____

    _____

20. How should you identify a resident before placing a meal tray?

    _____

    _____

    _____

    _____

Fill in the Blank

Choking

21. Choking can occur while eating, _____, or swallowing _____.

22. People who are weak, ill, or unconscious may choke on their own _____.

23. Residents should eat while sitting as _____ as possible.

24. Residents who have trouble _____ may have special diets.

25. Liquids that are _____ are easier to swallow.

Short Answer

Poisoning

26. List five things in a facility that can cause poisoning.

    _____

    _____

    _____

Name: _____

_____
_____
_____
_____

27. Which residents are especially vulnerable to poisoning?

_____
_____
_____
_____
_____

True or False

Cuts/Scrapes

28. ____ Cuts most often occur in the bedroom.

29. ____ Always put sharp objects away immediately after use.

30. ____ A wheelchair may be pushed in front of you or pulled behind you.

31. ____ When riding in an elevator with a resident in a wheelchair, you should turn the resident so that he faces the back of the elevator.

2. List safety guidelines for oxygen use

True or False

1. ____ Residents with breathing problems may receive oxygen that is more concentrated than what is in the air.

2. ____ Oxygen is prescribed by a doctor.

3. ____ Typically, nursing assistants adjust oxygen levels.

4. ____ Oxygen supports combustion; this means it makes other things burn.

5. ____ A flammable liquid like alcohol is fine to have in a room when oxygen is in use, as long as it is covered.

6. ____ It is all right to smoke in a room where oxygen is stored as long as the oxygen is not in use.

7. ____ Oxygen should be turned off in the event of a fire.

8. ____ Nursing assistants may administer oxygen if a resident specifically asks them to do so.

9. ____ It is important to check the skin around oxygen masks and tubing for irritation.

3. Explain the Material Safety Data Sheet (MSDS)

Multiple Choice

1. What is included on a Material Safety Data Sheet (MSDS)?
   (A) Chemical ingredients and dangers
   (B) Policy for reporting resident abuse
   (C) Form for reporting theft
   (D) Procedure for applying restraints

2. Employers must
   (A) Keep MSDS information confidential from employees
   (B) Terminate employees who do not know how to use an MSDS
   (C) Inform employees where MSDSs are kept
   (D) Destroy MSDSs if they do not agree with what is listed

4. Define the term "restraint" and give reasons why restraints were used

Multiple Choice

1. The purpose of restraints is
   (A) To discipline residents
   (B) To make the staff's job easier
   (C) To restrict voluntary movement or behavior
   (D) To allow residents to be left alone for longer periods

2. An example of a physical restraint is
   (A) A bed
   (B) A wheelchair
   (C) Medication
   (D) Side rails attached to a bed

3. A chemical restraint is
   (A) Medication used to control behavior
   (B) Medication used to treat illness
   (C) A medical procedure
   (D) A restraint tied to the person's ankles

4. What is one reason the use of restraints has been restricted?
   (A) They were found to be too expensive.
   (B) They were abused by caregivers.
   (C) They were difficult for caregivers to use.
   (D) They were not keeping residents occupied for a long enough period of time.

5. At the present time, restraints are used
   (A) For discipline
   (B) Only as a last resort
   (C) To stop residents from using call lights
   (D) Whenever the staff desires

5. List physical and psychological problems associated with restraints

Fill in the Blank

1. Reduced blood _____

2. Stress on the

   _____

3. Weakened

   _____

   and

   _____

4. _____

   sores

5. Risk of _____

6. Less _____,
   leading to poor appetite

7. _____

   disorders

8. Loss of _____
   and loss of

   _____

9. Severe

   _____ or

   even

   _____

6. Define the terms "restraint-free" and "restraint alternatives" and list examples of restraint alternatives

Multiple Choice

1. The law allows restraints to be used
   (A) When staff is too busy to properly care for residents
   (B) When residents do not like their roommates
   (C) Whenever a resident is depressed, agitated, or in a bad mood
   (D) When absolutely necessary for the safety of that person and others

2. "Restraint-free care" means that
   (A) Restraints are used when nurses request they be used
   (B) Restraints are used when necessary for safety
   (C) Restraints are never used for any reason
   (D) Restraints are used with permission from the resident's family

3. Restraint alternatives are
   (A) Any intervention used in place of a restraint or that reduces the need for a restraint
   (B) Any wrist or ankle restraint
   (C) Medications used to control a person's behavior
   (D) Periods of confining residents to their rooms

Short Answer

4. List five alternative actions that help reduce the need for a restraint.

   _____

   _____

   _____

   _____

   _____

   _____

   _____

7. Describe guidelines for what must be done if a restraint is ordered

True or False

1. _____ It is not necessary to check for an order before applying restraints.

2. _____ Restraints should be tied to the side rails of the bed.

3. _____ To make sure a restraint is not too tight, you should place a flat, open hand between the resident and the restraint.

4. _____ The call light should always be within reach of the resident.

5. _____ A resident who has a restraint applied must be checked every 30-60 minutes.

6. _____ At regular intervals, the restraint must be released or discontinued, and the resident must be offered help with toileting and offered fluids.

8. Explain the principles of body mechanics

True or False

1. _____ Back injury is a great risk that nursing assistants face.

2. _____ Using proper body mechanics can help you save energy and prevent injury.

3. _____ When lifting or carrying objects, you should hold them far away from your body.

4. _____ You should always point your feet in the direction in which you are moving.

5. _____ Keeping your feet close together gives your body the best base of support and keeps you more stable.

6. _____ It is best to rest objects against your forearm while lifting.

7. _____ A high center of gravity will give you a more stable base of support.

8. _____ You should always bend your knees when lifting an object.

9. Apply principles of body mechanics to daily activities

Scenario

Sharon is lifting a large box of supplies from the floor to place on a cart. Keeping her feet together, Sharon bends her knees and uses the muscles in her thighs, upper arms, and shoulders to lift the box. She holds the box at arm's length to place it on the cart. She is careful to move the box and her body at the same time while lifting.

1. What did Sharon do correctly? What should she have done differently?

_____

_____

_____

_____

_____

_____

_____

Fill in the Blank

2. Do not _____ when you are moving an object; always

_____

the object or person you are moving.

3. When lifting a heavy object from the floor, spread your feet

_____ apart.
_____ your knees.

4. Never try to "_____"
a falling resident. If the resident falls, assist her to the _____.

5. Bend your knees to lower yourself, rather than bending from the

_____.

6. If you are making an adjustable bed, adjust the height to a safe working level, usually

_____ high.

7. _____, slide, or pull objects rather than lifting them.

Name: _____

8. Hold objects _____
    to you when you are lifting or carrying them.

9. Get _____
    when possible for lifting or helping
    residents.

10. When moving a resident, let him know what
    you will do so he can help if possible.
    _____
    to three. Lift or move on three so everyone
    moves together.

10. Identify major causes of fire and list fire safety guidelines

Multiple Choice

1. What is needed for a fire to occur?
    (A) Heat
    (B) Water
    (C) Ice
    (D) Dirt

2. What is your first concern if a fire occurs?
    (A) Getting residents to safety
    (B) Putting out the fire
    (C) Saving important documentation
    (D) Saving expensive equipment

Fill in the Blank
Use the list of fire hazards in facilities to fill in the blanks below.

3. Careless _____
    or cigarettes left burning

4. Frayed or exposed
    _____ wires

5. _____ use

6. _____ liquids

7. Overloaded electrical _____

Short Answer

8. Explain the acronym for using a fire
    extinguisher.

    _____

    _____

    _____

    _____

    _____

    _____

    _____

9. Explain the acronym for response to fire.

    _____

    _____

    _____

    _____

    _____

10. Explain the fire safety technique "stop, drop,
    and roll."

    _____

    _____

    _____

    _____

    _____

7

Emergency Care and Disaster Preparation

1. Demonstrate how to recognize and respond to medical emergencies

Crossword

Across

1. If the person is unable to respond after you have asked him what has happened, he may be _____.

5. If the injured person is frightened, _____ to him and tell him what actions are being taken to help him.

8. Make sure you are not in _____ before you try to determine what has happened.

10. After an emergency, report the _____ only.

Down

2. When you come upon an emergency situation, remain calm, act quickly, and _____ clearly.

3. Notice the _____ when assessing the situation.

4. Once the emergency is over, you will have to file an _____ report.

6. Falls, _____, and cuts can be emergencies when they are severe.

7. If there is no response from the victim, call for _____ right away or send someone else to call.

9. Be _____ and confident to help reassure the injured person that he is being taken care of.

2. Demonstrate knowledge of CPR and first aid procedures

True or False

1. _____ CPR is an important skill for nursing assistants to learn.

2. _____ You should perform CPR on an unconscious victim even if you are not properly trained.

3. _____ You can contact the American Heart Association to schedule CPR training.

4. _____ Performing CPR incorrectly cannot further injure a person.

Name: _____

5. _____ Brain damage will not occur until 20 minutes after the heart stops beating and the lungs stop breathing.

6. _____ To check whether the person is responsive you should tap the person on the shoulder and shout, "Are you all right?"

7. _____ The person should be on his back on a hard surface (if he has no spinal injuries) before CPR is started.

8. _____ Look, listen, and feel for signs of life. If you do not detect adequate breathing within 60 seconds, give two rescue breaths.

9. _____ When giving rescue breaths, blow very deep breaths into the person's mouth.

10. _____ To give a chest compression, you should push in two inches with each compression.

Multiple Choice

11. What should you do if a resident needs CPR, but you are not trained to perform CPR?
    (A) Perform CPR anyway.
    (B) Perform CPR only with permission from the resident's family.
    (C) Perform CPR only if you think the victim will die if you do not.
    (D) Do not perform CPR.

12. What is the proper rate of chest compressions to rescue breaths when giving CPR?
    (A) 20 chest compressions to 1 rescue breath (20:1)
    (B) 30 chest compressions to 2 rescue breaths (30:2)
    (C) 15 chest compressions to 1 rescue breath (15:1)
    (D) 25 chest compressions to 2 rescue breaths (25:2)

13. How can you usually tell if a person is choking?
    (A) He will tell you.
    (B) He will ask for food.
    (C) He will put his hands to his throat and cough.
    (D) He will throw up.

14. After giving five back blows, if the object does not come out, where should you place your arms to give abdominal thrusts?
    (A) Under the person's arms and around his waist
    (B) Around his chest
    (C) Over his shoulders
    (D) Around his neck

15. How does a rescuer obtain consent to give a victim abdominal thrusts?
    (A) Rescuer asks victim's spouse to sign a consent form.
    (B) Rescuer asks facility administrator, "May I treat this resident who lives at your facility?"
    (C) Rescuer asks a lawyer.
    (D) Rescuer asks victim, "Are you choking? I know what to do. Can I help you?"

16. Signs of shock include
    (A) Pale or bluish skin
    (B) Lack of thirst
    (C) Happiness
    (D) Relaxation

17. If you suspect that a resident is having a heart attack, you should
    (A) Give him something cold to drink
    (B) Loosen the clothing around his neck
    (C) Encourage him to walk around
    (D) Leave him alone to rest

18. To control bleeding, you should
    (A) Use your bare hands to stop it
    (B) Lower the wound below the heart
    (C) Hold a thick pad or clean cloth against the wound and press down hard
    (D) Give the resident an aspirin for the pain

19. Which of the following is a common treatment for accidental poisoning?
    (A) Ibuprofen
    (B) Ginger root
    (C) Decongestant
    (D) Ipecac syrup

20. Which kind of burn involves just the outer layer of skin?
    (A) First degree
    (B) Second degree
    (C) Third degree
    (D) Freezer burn

21. To treat a minor burn, you should
    (A) Use ointment
    (B) Use grease, such as butter
    (C) Use ice water
    (D) Use cool, clean water

22. If a resident faints, you should
    (A) Lower him to the floor
    (B) Position him on his side
    (C) Elevate his legs one inch
    (D) Help him stand up immediately

23. If a resident has a nosebleed, what should be your first step?
    (A) Report and document the incident.
    (B) Apply pressure consistently until the bleeding stops.
    (C) Apply a cool cloth on the back of the neck, the forehead, or the upper lip.
    (D) Elevate the head of the bed or tell resident to remain in a sitting position.

24. When a resident is first experiencing signs of insulin reaction, what needs to happen?
    (A) Food that can be rapidly absorbed, such as hard candy, should be consumed.
    (B) The person should lie down and be left alone to rest.
    (C) The nursing assistant should give the resident medication.
    (D) CPR measures should be started immediately.

25. Which of the following is true about assisting a resident who is having a seizure?
    (A) Give the person a glass of water to drink.
    (B) Hold the person down if he or she is shaking severely.
    (C) Move furniture away to prevent injury to the person.
    (D) Open the person's mouth to move the tongue to the side.

26. Why is a quick response to a suspected stroke/CVA critical?
    (A) A quick response means that the family will not sue the facility.
    (B) Early treatment may be able to reduce the severity of the stroke.
    (C) Response time is not a factor in treating strokes.
    (D) Residents will experience no side effects at all if there is a quick response.

27. If a resident falls, you should
    (A) Wait until the end of the day to report the fall
    (B) Ask the resident to get up so that you can see if she can walk
    (C) Call for help
    (D) Move the resident to the bed

3. Describe disaster guidelines

Multiple Choice

1. A disaster kit should be assembled before disaster strikes. Disaster supplies include
   (A) An extra set of car keys and a change of clothing
   (B) A television set
   (C) Cosmetics and a hair dryer
   (D) Three pair of shoes

2. In a disaster, stay informed by
   (A) Running out to buy a newspaper
   (B) Going outside to find your friends
   (C) Listening to instructions from the nurse or administrator
   (D) Calling your psychic

3. If a disaster is forecast, be prepared by
   (A) Turning off your cell phone
   (B) Cleaning your house
   (C) Knowing how to start a fire
   (D) Wearing appropriate clothing and shoes

4. In the case of tornadoes, you should
   (A) Seek shelter inside, ideally in a steel-framed or concrete building
   (B) Hide close to the windows
   (C) Stay in a mobile home or trailer
   (D) Go outside so that you can see if the tornado is getting closer

5. In the case of lightning, you should
   (A) Find water and stay in the water
   (B) Stand by the largest tree you can find
   (C) Keep a metal object in your hand
   (D) Seek shelter in buildings

6. In the case of floods, you should
   (A) Fill the bathtub with fresh water
   (B) Drink water contaminated with flood water to stay hydrated
   (C) Handle electrical equipment
   (D) Turn off the gas by yourself

Name: _____

8

Human Needs and Human Development

1. Identify basic human needs

Short Answer

1. List six basic physical needs that all humans have.

_____

_____

_____

_____

_____

_____

2. List six psychosocial needs that humans have.

_____

_____

_____

_____

_____

_____

3. Complete your own hierarchy of needs below. Some of the examples have already been completed for you.

Maslow's Hierarchy of Needs

Need

(A) Need for self-actualization

(B) Need for self-esteem

(C) Need for love

(D) Safety and security needs

(E) Physical needs

Example

(A) I need the chance to learn new things.

(B) I need to know that I am doing a good job.

(C) _____

_____

(D) _____

_____

(E) _____

_____

2. Define "holistic care" and explain its importance in health care

Short Answer

In your own words, briefly define holistic care.

_____

_____

_____

_____

_____

_____

_____

_____

_____

_____

_____

3. Explain why independence and self-care are important

Short Answer

1. What is the greatest loss that you think you would experience if you had to move into a facility to live?

    _____

    _____

    _____

    _____

    _____

2. How do you think you would feel if you suddenly needed help with your ADLs?

    _____

    _____

    _____

    _____

    _____

3. List three self-care tasks that you will encourage residents to do for themselves.

    _____

    _____

    _____

    _____

4. List five problems that a loss of independence can cause.

    _____

    _____

    _____

    _____

    _____

4. Explain ways to accommodate sexual needs

True or False

1. ____ Sexual urges end as people get older.

2. ____ Ability to engage in sexual activity continues unless disease or injury occurs.

3. ____ Residents have the legal right to choose how to express their sexuality.

4. ____ All elderly people have the same sexual behavior and desires.

5. ____ If a person is unable to meet his sexual needs due to a disability, he will no longer have sexual desires.

6. ____ People who are confined to wheelchairs cannot have intimate relationships.

7. ____ Lack of privacy is a major reason for lack of sexual expression in long-term care facilities.

8. ____ You should always knock and wait for a response before entering residents' rooms.

9. ____ If you see a sexual encounter between residents, you should tell them to stop.

10. ____ If you encounter a resident being sexually abused, you should take him or her to a safe place and then notify the nurse.

Matching
Use each letter only once.

11. ____ One who wishes to be accepted as a member of the opposite sex

12. ____ A person who desires persons of both sexes

13. ____ A man whose sexual orientation is to other men

14. ____ A woman whose sexual orientation is to other women

15. ____ A person who has desire for persons of the opposite sex

(A) "Gay" or homosexual

(B) "Straight" or heterosexual

(C) Lesbian

(D Bisexual

(E) Transsexual

5. Identify ways to help residents meet their spiritual needs

Mark an "X" next to examples of appropriate ways to assist residents with their spiritual needs.

1. _____ A resident tells you that he cannot drink milk with his hamburger due to his religious beliefs. He asks you for some water instead. You take the milk away and bring him some water.

2. _____ A resident tells you she is a Baptist and wants to know if you will call the local Baptist church to find out when the next service will be. "A Baptist?" you ask. "Why don't you just attend a Catholic service instead? I'm a Catholic and my church is close by."

3. _____ A resident asks you to read a passage from his Bible. He tells you that it will comfort him. You open the Bible and begin to read.

4. _____ A resident wants to see a rabbi. You call the rabbi he wants to see.

5. _____ You see a Buddha statue in a resident's bedroom. You chuckle and tell the resident, "This is kind of funny-looking."

6. _____ A spiritual leader is visiting with a resident. You quietly leave the room and shut the door.

7. _____ A resident tells you he is Muslim. You begin to explain Christianity to him and ask him to attend a service at your church just to see what it is like.

8. _____ A resident tells you that she does not believe in God. You do believe in God but do not argue with her. You listen quietly as she tells you her reasons.

6. Identify ways to accommodate cultural and religious differences

Fill in the Blank
For each sentence, choose the correct term by using the words below. Some words may be used more than once.

Agnostics	Confucianism
Atheists	Hinduism
Buddhism	Islam
Christianity	Judaism

1. Worship at mosques

   _____

2. Religion practiced mostly in China and Japan

   _____

3. Take communion as a symbol of Christ's sacrifice

   _____

4. Believe that Allah (God) wants men to follow the teachings of the prophet Mohammed in the Koran

   _____

5. Religious leaders may be called priests, ministers, pastors, or deacons

   _____

6. Believe that God gave them laws through Moses and in the Bible, and that these laws should order their lives

   _____

7. Pray five times a day facing Mecca

   _____

8. This religion is based on the teachings of Siddhartha Gautama

   _____

9. May not do certain things, such as work or drive, on the Sabbath

   _____

10. Believe Jesus Christ was the son of God and that he died so their sins would be forgiven

    _____

Name: _____

11. Follow the teachings of the Vedas and Upanishads and believe in reincarnation

_____

12. Religious leaders are called rabbis

_____

13. People who do not deny that God might exist, but feel there is no true knowledge of God's existence

_____

14. People who claim that there is no God

_____

7. Describe the need for activity

Crossword

Across

4. Activity improves mood and

_____ .

5. Activity improves the ability to cope with

_____ .

8. Activity lessens the risk of

_____

disease and colon cancer.

9. Activity increases

_____ .

Down

1. Activity relieves symptoms of

_____ .

2. Activity also lessens the risk of diabetes and

_____ .

3. Activity lowers risk of

_____ .

5. Activity improves

_____

quality.

6. Activity increases appetite and promotes better _____
habits.

7. Activity improves _____
function.

8. Discuss family roles and their significance in health care

Multiple Choice
Read each description of residents' family lives below. Choose the term that best describes the kind of family they are from.

1. Mr. Dane's wife died giving birth to their twin girls. Mr. Dane never remarried and raised the girls himself.
   (A) Single-parent family
   (B) Nuclear family
   (C) Blended family
   (D) Multigenerational family

2. Ms. Cone has lived with her best friend, Ms. Lawrence, since they graduated from college together. They both dated many men throughout their lives but were never married. Ms. Cone has a teenage daughter who was raised in their household.
   (A) Single-parent family
   (B) Nuclear family
   (C) Blended family
   (D) Extended family

3. Mrs. Rose had three children with her first husband. She divorced him when their youngest child was two years old. Two years later she remarried, and she and her second husband raised her three children as well as one child from his first marriage.
   (A) Single-parent family
   (B) Nuclear family
   (C) Blended family
   (D) Multigenerational family

4. Mrs. Parker was married to her husband for thirty years. They lived together with their two children.
   (A) Single-parent family
   (B) Nuclear family
   (C) Blended family
   (D) Extended family

5. Mr. Potter was married in his twenties. He and his wife moved in with her parents and had three children. Later, when his younger sister was divorced, she also moved in with them.
   (A) Single-parent family
   (B) Nuclear family
   (C) Blended family
   (D) Multigenerational family

6. How is the family of today defined?
   (A) By blood relations
   (B) By how children are raised
   (C) By formal marriages
   (D) By support of one another

9. List ways to respond to emotional needs of residents and their families

True or False

1. _____ If a resident or family member comes to you with a problem or need, try to understand how he or she feels.

2. _____ If you simply sit quietly and listen when a resident tells you about a problem, he will think you do not care.

3. _____ Families may seek out nursing assistants because they are the closest staff members to the residents.

4. _____ You should spend all of your time focusing on the residents themselves, not their families.

5. _____ Using clichés is a good way to comfort residents.

6. _____ If you feel you cannot help a resident or family member, refer him to another qualified member of the care team.

10. Describe the stages of human growth and development and identify common disorders for each group

Infancy, Birth to 12 Months

True or False

1. _____ A child takes three years from birth to be able to move around, communicate basic needs, and feed himself.

2. _____ Infants develop from the hands to the head.

3. _____ Caregivers should encourage infants to stand as soon as they can hold their heads up.

4. _____ Studies show that putting an infant to sleep on its back can reduce the risk of sudden infant death syndrome (SIDS).

Short Answer

5. List three common disorders of infancy.

_____

_____

_____

_____

_____

_____

_____

_____

_____

Childhood

True or False

6. _____ Tantrums are common among toddlers.

7. _____ The best way to deal with tantrums is to give the toddler what he wants.

8. _____ Preschool children are too young to know right from wrong.

9. _____ Children aged 3 to 6 learn to speak.

10. _____ From the ages of 6 to 8 years, most children begin to go through puberty.

11. _____ School-age children (6 to 12 years) develop cognitively and socially.

Short Answer

12. List three common disorders of childhood.

_____

_____

_____

_____

_____

_____

Adolescence

True or False

13. _____ Puberty is the stage of growth when secondary sex characteristics, such as body hair, appear.

14. _____ Most adolescents do not struggle with peer acceptance, self-image or self-esteem.

15. _____ Adolescents may be moody due to changing hormones and peer pressure.

16. _____ Eating disorders cannot be life-threatening.

17. _____ Due to changes they are experiencing, adolescents may become depressed and may attempt suicide.

Short Answer

18. List three common disorders of adolescence.

_____

_____

_____

_____

_____

_____

Adulthood

True or False

19. _____ By eighteen years of age, most young adults have stopped developing physically, psychologically, and socially.

20. _____ One developmental task that most young adults undertake is to choose an occupation or career.

21. _____ A "mid-life crisis" is a period of unrest when a person has an unconscious desire for change and fulfillment of unmet goals.

22. _____ Middle adults usually do not experience any physical changes due to aging.

23. _____ Menopause is a condition that occurs in young women when the ovaries begin to secrete hormones.

24. _____ By the time a person reaches late adulthood, he or she must adjust to the effects of aging.

11. Distinguish between what is true and what is not true about the aging process

True or False

1. _____ Older adults have different capabilities depending upon their health.

2. _____ As people age, they often become lonely, forgetful, and slow.

3. _____ Diseases and illness are not a normal part of aging.

4. _____ Many older adults can lead active and healthy lives.

5. _____ Prejudice against older people is as unfounded and unfair as prejudice against racial, ethnic, or religious groups.

6. _____ Television and movies often present a false image of older adults.

7. _____ Skin becomes drier and less elastic with age.

8. _____ Responses and reflexes quicken as a person ages.

9. _____ Appetite increases with age.

10. _____ Urinary elimination becomes less frequent in older adults.

11. _____ Immunity weakens as a normal part of aging.

12. _____ Depression is normal in the elderly.

13. _____ Incontinence and loss of ability to think logically are not normal changes of aging. They should be reported to the nurse right away.

12. Explain developmental disabilities and list care guidelines

Multiple Choice

1. The four degrees of mental retardation are mild, moderate, severe, and _____.
   (A) Independent
   (B) Prolonged
   (C) Profound
   (D) Physical

2. In which of the following ways can nursing assistants help a developmentally disabled resident?
   (A) By teaching the resident how to drive
   (B) By performing all of the resident's ADLs
   (C) By teaching the resident self-care and assisting with ADLs
   (D) By ignoring the individual needs of the resident

Matching
Each letter may be used more than once.

3. _____ The most common developmental disorder

4. _____ May cause lack of control of the head, arms, and hands

5. _____ Complications may cause brain damage

6. _____ Causes different degrees of mental retardation, along with physical symptoms

7. _____ Caused by brain damage while in the uterus or during birth

8. _____ Sufferers develop at a below-average rate and may have below-average mental functioning

9. _____ Caused by part of the backbone not being well-developed at birth

10. _____ Causes a small skull, flattened nose, and shorter fingers

(A) Mental retardation

(B) Spina bifida

(C) Cerebral palsy

(D) Down syndrome

13. Identify community resources available to help the elderly

Short Answer

List five community resources available to the elderly.

_____

_____

_____

_____

_____

_____

Name: _____

9

The Healthy Human Body

1. Describe body systems and define key anatomical terms

Matching
Each letter may be used more than once.

1. _____ The body's building blocks

2. _____ Make up the systems of the body

3. _____ The body's physical and chemical processes

4. _____ Each has a specific function in the body

5. _____ Condition in which all body systems are working their best

6. _____ Make up the organs of the body

7. _____ Made up of groups of cells that perform similar tasks

(A) Homeostasis

(B) Metabolism

(C) Organs

(D) Tissues

(E) Cells

2. Describe the integumentary system

Fill in the Blank

1. The largest organ and system in the body is the _____.

2. Skin prevents _____ to internal organs.

3. Skin also prevents the loss of too much _____, which is essential to life.

4. The skin is also a _____ organ that feels heat, cold, pain, touch, and pressure.

5. Blood vessels _____, or widen, when the outside temperature is too high.

6. Blood vessels _____, or narrow, when the outside temperature is too cold.

Normal or Symptom
Determine which of the following are a normal part of the aging process and which are symptoms that need to be reported to the nurse. Write an "N" for normal aging and an "S" for a symptom to report.

7. _____ Thinning skin

8. _____ Bruises

9. _____ Cuts or wounds

10. _____ Wrinkles

11. _____ Brown spots

12. _____ Thinning of fatty tissue

13. _____ Rashes or flaking of skin

14. _____ Thinning or graying hair

15. _____ Less elastic skin

16. _____ Color changes in skin

17. _____ Swelling

18. _____ Drier skin

19. _____ "Orange-peel" look of skin

3. Describe the musculoskeletal system

True or False

1. ____ The body is shaped by muscles, bones, ligaments, tendons, and cartilage.

2. ____ The human body has 215 bones.

3. ____ Bones are made up of dead cells.

4. ____ Bones protect the body's organs.

5. ____ Two bones meet at a joint.

6. ____ A hinge joint, such as the elbow, can bend in two directions.

7. ____ Muscles allow movement of body parts.

8. ____ Skeletal muscles are involuntary muscles.

9. ____ The heart is an involuntary muscle.

10. ____ Range of motion exercises help prevent problems related to immobility.

11. ____ Atrophy occurs when the muscle weakens, decreases in size, and wastes away.

12. ____ Falls can be prevented by keeping paths clear and keeping walkers or canes in easy reach.

Normal or Symptom
Determine which of the following are a normal part of the aging process and which are symptoms that need to be reported to the nurse. Write an "N" for normal aging and an "S" for a symptom to report.

13. ____ Bruising

14. ____ Weakening of muscles

15. ____ Loss of muscle tone

16. ____ Change in ability to do routine movements or ROM exercises

17. ____ Loss of bone density

18. ____ Increased brittleness of bones

19. ____ Aches and pains

20. ____ Loss of height

21. ____ Pain during movement

22. ____ Increased swelling of joints

23. ____ White, shiny, warm, or red areas over a joint

24. ____ Slowing of body movement

4. Describe the nervous system

Multiple Choice

1. The nervous system
   (A) Gives the body shape and structure
   (B) Controls and coordinates body function
   (C) Is the largest organ in the body
   (D) Pumps blood through the blood vessels to the cells

2. The basic unit of the nervous system is
   (A) Neuron
   (B) Message
   (C) Brain
   (D) Spinal cord

3. The two main parts of the nervous system are
   (A) Cardiovascular system and integument
   (B) Neurons and receptors
   (C) The body and the brain
   (D) Central nervous system and peripheral nervous system

4. The central nervous system (CNS) is made up of
   (A) The brain and spinal cord
   (B) Muscles and bones
   (C) Neurons and receptors
   (D) Heart and lungs

5. The peripheral nervous system (PNS) deals with the outer part of the body using
   (A) The brain
   (B) Cerebrum
   (C) Nerves
   (D) Right hemisphere

6. What cushions the brain and spinal cord against injury?
   (A) The skull
   (B) The spinal column
   (C) The brain stem
   (D) Cerebrospinal fluid

7. The _____ is the part of the brain that controls thinking, speech, and voluntary muscles.
   (A) Brain stem
   (B) Cerebellum
   (C) Cerebral cortex
   (D) Right hemisphere

8. The left hemisphere of the brain controls
   (A) The left side of the body
   (B) The right side of the body
   (C) Both sides of the body
   (D) Memory

9. The brainstem controls
   (A) Smooth movements
   (B) Breathing and swallowing
   (C) Jerky movements
   (D) Emotions

10. The nerve pathways in the spinal cord conduct messages between
   (A) The heart and the blood
   (B) The cerebrum and cerebellum
   (C) The brain and the body
   (D) The muscles

Normal or Symptom
Determine which of the following are a normal part of the aging process and which are symptoms that need to be reported to the nurse. Write an "N" for normal aging and an "S" for a symptom to report.

11. _____ Inability to move one side of the body

12. _____ Depression or mood changes

13. _____ Fatigue or pain with movement

14. _____ Shaking

15. _____ Decreased sense of heat and cold

16. _____ Inability to speak clearly

17. _____ Decreased ability to perform ADLs

18. _____ Slower responses and reflexes

19. _____ Trouble swallowing

20. _____ Confusion

21. _____ Decreased sensitivity of nerve endings in skin

22. _____ Violent behavior

23. _____ Minor short-term memory loss

24. _____ Changes in vision or hearing

Short Answer

Sense Organs

25. List the five sense organs of the body.

   _____

   _____

   _____

   _____

   _____

26. Which part of the eye sends a message to the brain so that you can see?

   _____

   _____

   _____

   _____

27. List the three parts of the ear.

   _____

   _____

   _____

5. Describe the cardiovascular system

Fill in the Blank

1. The cardiovascular system is made up of the _____, blood, and blood _____.

2. The blood carries food, _____, and other substances to the body.

3. If circulation is reduced, _____ products of cell metabolism build up in the blood.

4. _____ is the liquid portion of the blood.

5. Red blood cells are produced by bone _____.

6. Blood gets its red color from _____.

7. _____ blood cells defend the body against foreign substances.

8. _____ cause the blood to clot to stop excess bleeding.

9. The three layers of the heart muscle are the _____, the myocardium, and the endocardium.

10. The upper _____ of the heart are called the left and right _____.

11. Two _____ allow the blood to flow in only one direction.

12. The _____ is the resting phase of the heart.

13. The _____ is the contracting phase of the heart.

14. _____ carry oxygen-rich blood away from the heart.

15. _____ carry the blood containing waste products from the capillaries back to the heart.

Normal or Symptom
Determine which of the following are a normal part of the aging process and which are symptoms that need to be reported to the nurse. Write an "N" for normal aging and an "S" for a symptom to report.

16. ____ Severe headache

17. ____ Heart pumps less efficiently

18. ____ Chest pain

19. ____ Swelling of hands or feet

20. ____ Changes in pulse rate

21. ____ Pale or bluish hands or feet

22. ____ Fatigue

23. ____ Shortness of breath

6. Describe the respiratory system

True or False

1. ____ Respiration occurs in the lungs.

2. ____ Expiration is breathing in.

3. ____ The respiratory system brings oxygen into the body and removes carbon dioxide.

4. ____ The larynx is also called the windpipe.

5. ____ Oxygen and carbon dioxide are exchanged between the alveoli and the capillaries.

6. ____ The pleura is a membrane that covers the lungs.

7. ____ Regular exercise and deep breathing should be encouraged.

Normal or Symptom
Determine which of the following are a normal part of the aging process and which are symptoms that need to be reported to the nurse. Write an "N" for normal aging and an "S" for a symptom to report.

8. ____ Decreased lung strength and capacity

9. ____ Discolored sputum

10. ____ Need to sit after mild exertion

11. ____ Shallow breathing

12. ____ Pale or bluish lips, arms, or legs

13. ____ Weaker voice

14. ____ Coughing or wheezing

15. ____ Nasal congestion

16. ____ Change in respiratory rate

7. Describe the urinary system

Short Answer

1. List the two vital functions of the urinary system.

_____

_____

_____

_____

Name: _____

2. Why are women more likely to suffer from urinary tract infections than men?

_____
_____
_____
_____

3. How should you respond to urinary incontinence?

_____
_____
_____
_____

Normal or Symptom
Determine which of the following are a normal part of the aging process and which are symptoms that need to be reported to the nurse. Write an "N" for normal aging and an "S" for a symptom to report.

4. ____ Pain during urination
5. ____ Bladder does not empty completely
6. ____ Bladder feels full or painful
7. ____ Pain in kidney region
8. ____ Changes in color of urine
9. ____ Urinary incontinence
10. ____ Swelling in extremities

8. Describe the gastrointestinal system

Crossword
Fill in the blanks below and use your answers to complete the crossword puzzle.

Across

2. _____ is semi-solid material made up of water, solid waste material, bacteria, and mucus that passes through the rectum and out of the body.

7. The esophagus moves food into the stomach through involuntary contractions called _____.

8. Feces move out of the body through the _____, the rectal opening.

Down

1. The GI system is made up of the _____ tract and other digestive organs.

3. The digestive process turns food into _____, a semi-liquid substance.

4. _____ should fit properly and be cleaned regularly.

5. _____, a green liquid produced by the liver, helps break down dietary fat.

6. The functions of the gastrointestinal system are digestion and _____.

Normal or Symptom
Determine which of the following are a normal part of the aging process and which are symptoms that need to be reported to the nurse. Write an "N" for normal aging and an "S" for a symptom to report.

9. ____ Flatulence
10. ____ Decrease in saliva
11. ____ Anorexia
12. ____ Abnormally-colored stool

Name: _____

13. _____ Anal incontinence

14. _____ Decreased absorption of nutrients

15. _____ Diarrhea

16. _____ Less efficient digestion

17. _____ Heartburn

9. Describe the endocrine system

Matching
Each letter is used only once.

1. _____ Causes the uterus to contract during childbirth

2. _____ Master gland of the body

3. _____ Controls the balance of fluids in the body

4. _____ Produces hormones that regulate the ability to reproduce

5. _____ Secretes a hormone to regulate calcium use

6. _____ Secretes insulin

7. _____ Regulates the amount of sugar (glucose) available to the cells for metabolism

8. _____ Produces hormones that regulate salt and water absorption in kidneys and produce the hormone adrenaline

9. _____ Located in the neck in front of the larynx and produces thyroid hormone

(A) Pancreas

(B) Pituitary gland

(C) Thyroid gland

(D) Antidiuretic hormone

(E) Insulin

(F) Parathyroid glands

(G) Oxytocin

(H) Adrenal glands

(I) Gonads

Normal or Symptom
Determine which of the following are a normal part of the aging process and which are symptoms that need to be reported to the nurse. Write an "N" for normal aging and an "S" for a symptom to report.

10. _____ Excessive perspiration

11. _____ Dizziness

12. _____ Hyperactivity

13. _____ Blurred vision

14. _____ Less able to handle stress

15. _____ Irritability

16. _____ Headache

17. _____ Reduced insulin production

18. _____ Hunger

19. _____ Decrease in hormone levels

20. _____ Confusion

21. _____ Weakness

10. Describe the reproductive system

Multiple Choice

1. The reproductive system allows humans to
   (A) Move and speak
   (B) Create human life
   (C) Think logically
   (D) Fight disease

2. The hormone needed for male reproductive organs to function properly is
   (A) Sperm
   (B) Adrenaline
   (C) Estrogen
   (D) Testosterone

3. The tube through which males pass both urine and semen is called the
   (A) Prostate
   (B) Penis
   (C) Urethra
   (D) Seminal vesicle

4. The gonads in human females are called
   (A) Ovaries
   (B) Eggs
   (C) Testicles
   (D) Sex cells

5. The female reproductive cycle is maintained by the hormones
(A) Estrogen and progesterone
(B) Adrenaline and progesterone
(C) Testosterone and ADH
(D) Insulin and testosterone

6. The _____ contains blood vessels to provide for the growth of an embryo.
(A) Endometrium
(B) Uterus
(C) Fallopian tube
(D) Fundus

7. A baby develops inside the
(A) Endometrium
(B) Cervix
(C) Fallopian tube
(D) Fundus

Normal or Symptom

Determine which of the following are a normal part of the aging process and which are symptoms that need to be reported to the nurse. Write an "N" for normal aging and an "S" for a symptom to report.

8. ____ Impotence (male)

9. ____ Decrease in estrogen (female)

10. ____ Swelling of genitals

11. ____ Enlarged prostate gland (male)

12. ____ End of menstruation (female)

13. ____ Discharge from penis or vagina

14. ____ Blood in urine or stool

15. ____ Painful intercourse

16. ____ Decrease in sperm production (male)

17. ____ Sores on genitals

18. ____ Discomfort with urination

11. Describe the immune and lymphatic systems

Fill in the Blank

1. The immune system protects the body from disease-causing _____, viruses, and _____.

2. _____ immunity protects the body from disease in general.

3. _____ immunity protects against a disease that is invading the body at a given time.

4. _____ barriers, such as the skin and _____ membranes, are a physical barrier against invaders.

5. Body temperature and the acidity of some organs are _____ barriers against infection.

6. The ability to fight infection through the swelling of an area is an _____ response.

7. When an invader has been eliminated, the body records the event in the form of _____. This prevents the disease from threatening the body again.

8. _____ immunity is obtained through fighting infection or by vaccination.

9. The lymphatic system removes extra _____ and _____ products from the tissues.

10. _____ is a clear yellow fluid that carries disease-fighting cells. The cells are called _____.

11. When the body is fighting infection, _____ may occur in the lymph nodes.

12. Lymph fluid is circulated by _____ activity, massage, and _____.

Name: _____

Normal or Symptom

Determine which of the following are a normal part of the aging process and which are symptoms that need to be reported to the nurse. Write an "N" for normal aging and an "S" for a symptom to report.

13. _____ Swelling of lymph nodes

14. _____ Increased fatigue

15. _____ Decreased response to vaccines

16. _____ Increased risk of infection

10

Positioning, Lifting, and Moving

1. Review the principles of body mechanics

Fill in the Blank

1. _____
   the load. Decide if you can move it safely without
   _____.

2. Think ahead, _____
   and _____
   the move. Look for any potential
   _____.

3. Check your base of
   _____.
   Be sure you have firm
   _____.

4. Face what you are
   _____.

5. Keep your back
   _____.

6. Begin in a
   _____
   position. Bend at the hips and
   _____.

7. Tighten your
   _____
   muscles when starting the lift.

8. Keep the object
   _____
   to your body. Lift objects to the level of your
   _____.

9. _____
   or _____
   when you can rather than lifting.

2. Explain beginning and ending steps in care procedures

Word Search
Fill in the blanks below and find your answers in the word search.

Beginning Steps

1. _____
   your hands. This is the best way to prevent infection.

2. _____
   yourself and the resident by name.

3. Explain the
   _____
   to the resident. Maintain
   _____
   contact when possible.

4. Provide for
   _____
   with a curtain, screen, or door.

5. Adjust the bed to a safe
   _____.
   If it is movable,
   _____ the wheels.

Ending Steps

6. Make the resident
   _____.
   The bed should be free from
   _____
   and _____.

7. Return the bed to the lowest
   _____.

8. Place _____
   within resident's reach before leaving.

Name: _____

9. Wash your _____.

10. Report any

_____

in resident to the nurse.

11. _____

the procedure. Use

_____

guidelines.

```
t  h  u  y  a  e  n  v  s  k  c  o  l  y
h  a  f  x  t  q  r  e  l  o  s  o  f  c
g  n  g  l  w  i  g  u  m  x  r  h  y  a
i  d  z  a  e  n  l  f  d  y  u  f  h  v
l  s  s  g  a  v  o  i  v  e  i  m  o  i
l  h  p  h  h  r  e  r  c  t  c  k  f  r
l  m  c  i  t  p  w  l  n  a  n  o  n  p
a  e  c  a  f  o  t  e  c  a  f  k  r  i
c  k  b  n  w  s  d  c  r  u  m  b  s  p
w  l  g  u  d  i  w  r  i  n  k  l  e  s
e  h  p  f  t  t  n  e  m  u  c  o  d  a
w  b  g  p  l  i  y  g  b  u  v  y  z  c
t  r  l  b  j  o  v  h  s  x  a  x  y  j
i  v  u  d  e  n  z  k  m  c  x  w  n  u
```

3. Explain positioning and describe how to safely position residents

Multiple Choice

1. Why do residents who spend a lot of time in bed need repositioning at least every two hours?
   (A) They have their sheets changed that often at the same time.
   (B) They have a risk of skin breakdown and pressure sores.
   (C) They will need to be able to talk to visitors.
   (D) Their family members will sue the facility if they are not.

2. In this position the resident is lying on either side. The knee on the upper side of the body should be flexed.
   (A) Supine
   (B) Lateral
   (C) Prone
   (D) Fowler's

3. In this position, the resident is lying on the abdomen. This position is uncomfortable for many elderly people.
   (A) Sims'
   (B) Lateral
   (C) Prone
   (D) Fowler's

4. A draw sheet is used to
   (A) Make residents more comfortable
   (B) Help residents sleep more easily
   (C) Reposition residents without causing shearing
   (D) Prevent incontinence

5. Logrolling is
   (A) A way to measure bedbound residents' weight
   (B) A way to record vital signs
   (C) Moving a resident as a unit without disturbing alignment
   (D) A method of bedmaking

6. Dangling is
   (A) Lying in the supine position
   (B) Doing a few sit-ups in bed to get used to the upright position
   (C) Elevating the resident's feet with pillows
   (D) A way to help residents regain balance after lying down

7. A resident in the Fowler's position is
   (A) In a semi-sitting position (45 to 60 degrees)
   (B) Lying flat on his or her back
   (C) In a left side-lying position
   (D) Lying on his or her stomach

Labeling
Label each position below and describe comfort measures appropriate for each.

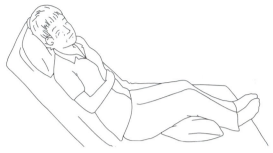

8. _____

Comfort measures: _____

_____

_____

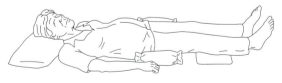

9. _____

Comfort measures: _____

_____

_____

10. _____

Comfort measures: _____

_____

_____

11. _____

Comfort measures: _____

_____

_____

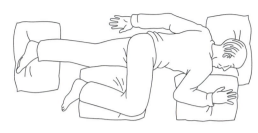

12. _____

Comfort measures: _____

_____

_____

4. Describe how to safely transfer residents

Multiple Choice

1. Which of the following statements is true of wheelchairs?
   (A) Before transferring a resident, make sure the wheelchair is unlocked and movable.
   (B) Check the resident's alignment in the chair after a transfer is complete.
   (C) To fold a standard wheelchair, turn it upside-down and make the seat flatten.
   (D) All residents will need you to transfer them to their wheelchairs.

2. Some residents have a stronger side and a weaker side. The weaker side of the body is called the
   (A) Released side
   (B) Separated side
   (C) Ambulated side
   (D) Involved or affected side

3. When applying a transfer (gait) belt, you should place it
   (A) Around the wheelchair's backrest
   (B) Underneath the resident's clothing, on bare skin
   (C) Over the resident's clothing and around the waist
   (D) Around your waist so the resident can hold onto it

Name: _____

4. The following piece of equipment may be used to help transfer residents who are unable to bear weight on their legs
   (A) Sling
   (B) Slide or transfer board
   (C) Wheeled table
   (D) Folded blanket

5. Which of the following statements is true of mechanical, or hydraulic, lifts?
   (A) You do not need to be trained to use mechanical lifts.
   (B) The legs of the stand need to be closed, in their narrowest position, before helping the resident into the lift.
   (C) Lifts help prevent injury to you and the resident.
   (D) These lifts are used to transport residents in the car.

6. When transferring residents who have a one-sided weakness, which side moves first?
   (A) Left side
   (B) Either side
   (C) Weaker side
   (D) Stronger side

7. If a resident starts to fall, the best thing to do is
   (A) Widen your stance, bend your knees, and lower the resident to the floor
   (B) Catch the resident under the arms to stop the fall
   (C) Move away and allow the resident to fall on her own
   (D) Let the resident fall on top of you to break the fall

5. Discuss how to safely ambulate residents

Multiple Choice

1. A resident who has some difficulty with balance but can bear weight on both legs should use a
   (A) Walker
   (B) Crutch
   (C) Wheelchair
   (D) Transfer board

2. Ambulation is another word for
   (A) Walking
   (B) Movement in a wheelchair
   (C) Riding in an ambulance
   (D) Logrolling

3. In addition to a transfer (gait) belt, what equipment should you have when you assist a resident to ambulate?
   (A) Mechanical lift
   (B) Rocking chair
   (C) Extra pillows
   (D) Non-skid shoes

4. When helping a visually-impaired resident walk, it is important to
   (A) Keep the resident in front of you
   (B) Let the resident walk beside and slightly behind you
   (C) Walk quickly
   (D) Avoid mentioning stepping up or down

5. Which of the following assistive devices for walking has four rubber-tipped feet?
   (A) C cane
   (B) Quad cane
   (C) Crutch
   (D) Gait belt

6. When using a cane, the resident should place it on his _____ side.
   (A) Left
   (B) Right
   (C) Weaker
   (D) Stronger

11

Admitting, Transferring, and Discharging

1. Describe how residents may feel when entering a facility

Short Answer

What makes moving to a facility a big adjustment for residents?

_____

_____

_____

_____

_____

_____

_____

_____

_____

_____

_____

_____

_____

_____

_____

2. Explain the nursing assistant's role in the admission process

Word Search
Fill in the blanks below and find your answers in the word search.

1. The first time you meet a new resident is often at

    _____.

2. Make sure a resident has a good

    _____
    of you and your facility.

3. Prepare the

    _____
    before the resident arrives.

4. Ask _____
    to find out a resident's personal preferences and

    _____.

5. _____
    yourself to the resident and state your position.

6. Always call a resident by his

    _____
    name until he tells you what he prefers to be called.

7. Make sure the new resident feels welcome and wanted. Never

    _____
    the process or the new resident.

8. Tell the resident about daily life in the facility and offer him a

    _____.

9. New residents must be given a

    _____
    copy of their rights.

10. It is important to

    _____
    the new resident's condition in order to recognize any changes that may take place later.

11. A resident has a legal

    _____
    to have his personal items treated carefully. Handle personal items with care and respect.

Name: _____

```
n l g t y c k j h o p f n w
n o i s s e r p m i c w t a
d h i n s r f o m k a v s h
q u e s t i o n s t e d s o
u l p e s r z q a q w u m k
e b w n n i o b s e r v e e
g a x i x g m d x h i n v b
l d j t h h y d u a t h c z
o a r u o t y o a c t o n q
c f m o u e p n s d e s q o
h k m r i g b d r n n m h g
s g f g o x l q c i o h m m
n i q e f f i w b z d j g r
i b l r x z y h v y f n j y
```

Short Answer

12. Why must any weight loss, no matter how small, be reported?

_____

_____

_____

_____

_____

3. Explain the nursing assistant's role during an in-house transfer of a resident

True or False

1. _____ A transfer to a new facility or a hospital is very easy for residents to handle.

2. _____ Residents should be informed of transfers as early as possible.

3. _____ The resident will usually pack her own belongings for a transfer.

4. _____ You should introduce the resident to everyone in the new area.

5. _____ Residents have the legal right to be notified in advance of a room or roommate change.

4. Explain the nursing assistant's role in the discharge of a resident

Scenario

1. Mr. Carpenter has been at the Green Garden Skilled Nursing Facility for six months to recover from a broken hip. He has made an excellent recovery. His doctor has written a discharge order, and he is now ready to return home. As you are packing his things for him, he tells you that he is afraid that he will not be able to take care of himself at home. What will you say to express your concern and reassure him?

_____

_____

_____

_____

_____

2. What are five things that the nurse will probably discuss with Mr. Carpenter and his family before he is discharged?

_____

_____

_____

_____

_____

_____

_____

_____

_____

5. Describe the nursing assistant's role in physical exams

Multiple Choice

1. What are the nursing assistant's duties during residents' physical exams?
   (A) Performing the exams
   (B) Giving injections
   (C) Diagnosing illness or disease
   (D) Getting equipment for the doctor or nurse

2. In which position is the resident placed for examination of the breasts, chest, and abdomen?
   (A) Dorsal recumbent
   (B) Lithotomy position
   (C) Knee-chest position
   (D) Trendelenburg position

3. Which of the following pieces of equipment is used to measure blood pressure?
   (A) Reflex hammer
   (B) Thermometer
   (C) Sphygmomanometer
   (D) Otoscope

Short Answer

4. List three responsibilities of a nursing assistant after a resident exam is completed.

   _____

   _____

   _____

   _____

   _____

   _____

   _____

   _____

   _____

   _____

5. List two rights of residents regarding exams.

   _____

   _____

   _____

   _____

   _____

   _____

   _____

12

The Resident's Unit

1. Explain why a comfortable environment is important for the resident's well-being

Word Search

Fill in the blanks in the statements below, then find your answers in the word search.

1. Common _____ in facilities can upset and/or irritate residents.

2. Do not _____ equipment or meal trays.

3. Keep your _____ low and _____ doors when residents ask you to.

4. Promptly clean up after episodes of _____. Change incontinence _____ as soon as they are soiled. Dispose of them properly.

5. Empty and clean bedpans, _____, commodes, and _____ basins right away.

6. Give regular oral care and _____ care to help avoid body and breath odors.

7. Due to loss of protective fatty tissue and illness, older residents may feel _____ often.

8. _____ clothes and bed covers for warmth. Keep residents _____ during personal care.

9. Good _____ promotes safety and helps prevent falls. Residents may prefer _____ rooms when they are ill or are sleeping.

```
e p l m e s f s v b j g e z
n c a c e q b r r r n o c n
a q n s w m l i e i j p i n
m b o e b g e r t k p l o o
j l s s n f j h r i r f v i
c v r b s i g u r i n a l s
c k e x a i t l a y e r d e
m o p n l n f n g j c z l s
n x v z p x g k o s z l c g
i u w e h i r e c c d w o v
l k k p r i f s n c n s l g
s i s e m e a r y s k i d n
x z o d t d d y p s q u p o
v k i v v c g f m h b n j d
```

2. Describe a standard resident unit

True or False

1. ____ A resident's room is his home and must be treated with respect.

2. ____ It is not necessary to wait for permission to enter a resident's room, as many residents will not be able to hear your knock.

3. ____ Normally, residents' beds are kept in their highest position.

4. ____ Urinals and bedpans may be stored inside the bedside stand.

5. ____ Urinals and bedpans may be stored on top of the overbed table.

6. ____ Call lights must always be answered promptly.

7. ____ Call lights should be placed wherever it is easiest for the nursing assistant to reach them.

Name: _____

8. ____ Privacy curtains block sight, as well as sound.

9. ____ Residents have a legal right to have their privacy protected when receiving care.

10. ____ Soiled linen should not be placed on an overbed table.

3. Discuss how to care for and clean unit equipment

Multiple Choice

1. If you are asked to use a piece of equipment you do not know how to work, you should
   (A) Figure it out as you go along
   (B) Try to perform the procedure without using the equipment
   (C) Ask for help
   (D) Refuse to use the equipment

2. Disposable equipment
   (A) Is used once and then discarded
   (B) Is used three times and then discarded
   (C) Is sterilized before it is reused
   (D) Is not used in care facilities

3. Before you leave a resident's room, you should
   (A) Adjust the room temperature so that you feel comfortable
   (B) Place the call light within the resident's reach
   (C) Rearrange the resident's items to make more space
   (D) Mop the resident's floor and clean her windows

4. Call lights should be placed
   (A) Within the nursing assistant's reach
   (B) Within the nurse's reach
   (C) Within the housekeeping staff's reach
   (D) Within the resident's reach

4. Explain the importance of sleep and factors affecting sleep

Short Answer

1. List five things that can disrupt a resident's sleep.

_____

_____

_____

_____

_____

_____

_____

_____

2. List three problems that can be caused by lack of sleep.

_____

_____

_____

_____

_____

_____

3. List four things that you should look for when a resident complains that he or she is not sleeping well.

_____

_____

_____

_____

_____

_____

_____

5. Describe bedmaking guidelines and perform proper bedmaking

Multiple Choice

1. Why is it important to change bed linens often?
   (A) To get residents out of their beds and to activities
   (B) To rotate clean sheets evenly
   (C) To keep NAs' skills up-to-date
   (D) To prevent infection and to promote comfort

2. Why should bed linens be carried away from your body?
   (A) To prevent contamination of your clothes
   (B) To keep the linens neat
   (C) To avoid mixing up the linens of different residents
   (D) For good body alignment

3. When removing dirty linen, you should
   (A) Fold it so that the dirtiest area is outside
   (B) Roll it so that the dirtiest area is inside
   (C) Gather it in a bunch
   (D) Shake it to remove particles

4. When a resident cannot get out of bed
   (A) The bed cannot be changed
   (B) The resident will be moved to a stretcher for bed changing
   (C) The nurse will change the bed
   (D) The bed should be raised to a safe height before you make it

5. Soiled linen should be bagged
   (A) In the hallway
   (B) In another resident's room
   (C) At the point of origin
   (D) At the nurses' station

6. A surgical bed is
   (A) A bed used during surgery
   (B) A bed made to easily accept residents returning on stretchers
   (C) A bed used for special personal care procedures
   (D) Any bed on a residential unit

7. A bed made with the bedspread and blankets in place is called a(n)
   (A) Open bed
   (B) Stretcher bed
   (C) Closed bed
   (D) Completed bed

Name: _____

13

Personal Care Skills

1. Explain personal care of residents

Crossword
Fill in the blanks below and use your answers to complete the crossword puzzle.

Across

3. Keep residents

   _____

   when possible while helping them dress.

4. Practices that maintain personal appearance and neatness, such as caring for fingernails and hair, are called

   _____.

6. Do not _____
   a resident when she is in the bathroom or is getting dressed.

7. Some residents will need more

   _____

   with personal care than others.

9. Observe residents' mental and

   _____

   state while assisting with personal care.

10. When assisting with personal care, always provide plenty of

    _____.

Down

1. _____
   is the term used to describe practices to keep bodies clean and healthy.

2. Assisting with a.m. care includes helping with mouth care before or after

   _____.

3. During personal care, observe for problems
   or _____
   that have occurred.

5. While assisting with personal care, encourage residents to care for themselves. Promoting

   _____

   is an important part of your care.

8. Before you begin a procedure,

   _____

   what you will be doing. Doing this is not only the resident's legal right, but it can also help lessen anxiety.

Name: _____

_____

_____

2. Identify guidelines for providing good skin care and preventing pressure sores

Short Answer

1. List the four accepted stages of pressure sores, including a brief description of what the sore looks like at each stage.

_____
_____
_____
_____
_____
_____
_____
_____
_____
_____
_____
_____
_____

2. List eight important observations to make about changes in a resident's skin.

_____
_____
_____
_____
_____
_____
_____
_____
_____
_____

3. What are three changes in ebony complexions that might indicate injury to the tissue?

_____
_____

Labeling

For each position shown, list the areas at risk for pressure sores.

Prone Position

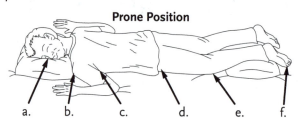

a.   b.   c.   d.   e.   f.

4. Prone Position
   a. _____
   b. _____
   c. _____
   d. _____
   e. _____
   f. _____

Supine Position

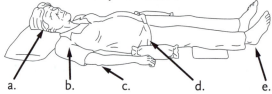

a.   b.   c.   d.   e.

5. Supine Position
   a. _____
   b. _____
   c. _____
   d. _____
   e. _____

Lateral Position

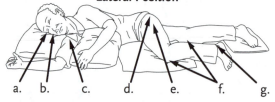

a. b. c. d. e. f. g.

6. Lateral Position
   a. _____
   b. _____
   c. _____
   d. _____
   e. _____
   f. _____
   g. _____

True or False

7. _____ When skin begins to break down, it becomes pale, white, or a reddened color.

8. _____ Immobile residents should be repositioned every four hours.

9. _____ Pressure sores usually occur in areas of the body where bone is close to the skin.

10. _____ If residents are seated in chairs or wheelchairs, they do not need to be repositioned.

11. _____ If NAs notice areas where the skin is red or purple, they should massage those areas.

12. _____ Proper nutrition helps keep the skin healthy.

13. _____ When transferring or positioning residents, pull them across the sheets to make the job easier.

14. _____ Another name for pressure sores is decubitus ulcers.

15. _____ Common sites for pressure sores are the chest, nose, and hands.

Matching
Use each letter only once.

16. _____ Placed against the feet to keep them properly aligned and to prevent foot drop

17. _____ Keeps bedcovers from pushing down on the feet

18. _____ Areas of the body where the bone lies close to the skin

19. _____ Used to help residents who cannot assist with turning or moving in bed; helps prevent skin damage from shearing

20. _____ Keeps fingers from curling tightly

21. _____ Keeps hips from turning outward

22. _____ Helps support and align a limb and improve its functioning (e.g., a splint)

23. _____ Areas of the body that bear much of its weight

(A) Footboard

(B) Pressure points

(C) Draw sheet

(D) Bony prominences

(E) Trochanter rolls

(F) Bed cradle

(G) Hand rolls

(H) Orthotic device

3. Explain guidelines for assisting with bathing

True or False

1. _____ Bathing promotes good health and helps prevent skin irritation and body odor.

2. _____ A partial bath includes washing the face, ears, and hair.

3. _____ The doctor and the resident decide which type of bath is appropriate for the resident.

4. _____ When washing a resident's eyes and face, use lots of soap on a wet washcloth.

5. _____ An additive is a substance added to another substance, changing its effect.

6. _____ The perineum should be washed every day.

7. _____ Older skin produces more perspiration than younger skin.

8. _____ The resident should test the temperature of the water before bathing because he or she is best able to choose a comfortable water temperature.

9. _____ When washing a female's perineal area, wipe from back to front.

10. _____ Residents should always be covered while going to and from the shower or tub room.

11. _____ Using bath oils during baths is helpful for residents with dry skin.

12. _____ Whirlpool baths help stimulate circulation and wound healing.

4. Explain guidelines for assisting with grooming

Short Answer

1. List one benefit of good grooming.

_____

_____

_____

_____

2. Describe two grooming routines that are important in your life. Why do you think routines are important to people even when they are ill?

_____

_____

_____

_____

_____

_____

_____

_____

3. Why should you never cut a resident's toenails?

_____

_____

_____

_____

_____

4. List eight observations that should be made about the feet when giving foot care.

_____

_____

_____

_____

_____

_____

_____

_____

_____

_____

_____

5. Why should you wear gloves while shaving residents?

_____

_____

_____

6. Why should electric razors not be used near any water, when oxygen is in use, or if a person has a pacemaker?

_____

_____

_____

_____

7. The textbook says, "Do not comb or brush residents' hair into a childish style." Why do you think this statement is included?

_____

_____

_____

_____

_____

8. What are ways that NAs can help prevent the spread of lice?

_____

_____

_____

_____

5. List guidelines for assisting with dressing

Word Search

1. Encourage residents to wear

_____
clothes, not nightclothes, during the day.

2. Provide _____
by covering the resident with a bath blanket, closing the door, and never exposing more than you need to.

3. For residents who have weakness or paralysis on one side, place the

_____
arm or leg through the garment first. When undressing, start with the

_____
side.

4. The resident's clothing for the day should be chosen by the

_____.

5. Clothing that is a size

_____

than the resident normally wears is easier to put on.

6. _____

bras are easier for female residents to work by themselves.

7. _____

aids or equipment are used to help with dressing and help maintain independence.

8. When putting on socks or stockings,

_____

or fold them down before slipping them over the toes and foot.

```
l y k s u w x w r u m t o c
r y t n e d i s e r x n g z
v z k b g b t o q a i m o f
g d l l o r u a g y k a d y
p w g t o v o d c o c e c b
g n i n e t s a f t n o r f
i i g f q b v p v u z b w u
r e x r k i w t m u x g a r
r z g m r z i i n i z f o a
k t t p j e w v z p s l k l
u v v c j p g e j h u u q u
h v g j p k v r w z c q d g
q d m v y l d i a d a i m e
r z r w z c k x s l a t p r
```

6. Identify guidelines for good oral care

Short Answer

1. How often should oral care be performed? When should it be done?

_____

_____

_____

_____

_____

2. How does performing proper, regular oral care help the mouth?

_____

_____

_____

_____

_____

_____

3. List eight signs to observe and report about the mouth when performing oral care.

_____

_____

_____

_____

_____

_____

_____

_____

_____

_____

_____

_____

4. What is aspiration? How can you help prevent aspiration during oral care of unconscious residents?

_____

_____

_____

_____

_____

_____

7. Define "dentures" and explain how to care for dentures

Multiple Choice

1. Dentures must be handled carefully because
   (A) A resident cannot eat without them
   (B) They do not cost much
   (C) A resident will look unattractive without them
   (D) A resident will sue for libel if they are broken

2. How should dentures be stored?
   (A) In a denture cup labeled with the resident's name and room number
   (B) At the nurse's station
   (C) Wrapped in a paper towel
   (D) In hot water

3. If you are removing a resident's dentures, the resident should be
   (A) Lying down on his back
   (B) Standing
   (C) Sitting upright
   (D) Lying down on his side

4. When inserting dentures
   (A) Apply antibiotic ointment to the dentures first
   (B) Use your bare hands
   (C) Apply powder, then warm water to get the dentures to stick
   (D) Place upper denture into the mouth by turning it at an angle

Name: _____

14

Basic Nursing Skills

1. Explain the importance of monitoring vital signs

Short Answer

1. What can changes in vital signs indicate?

_____

_____

2. Which changes should be immediately reported to a supervisor?

_____

_____

_____

_____

2. List guidelines for taking body temperature

Short Answer

1. What are the four sites for measuring body temperature?

_____

_____

_____

2. Name seven conditions that indicate you should not take the person's temperature orally.

_____

_____

_____

_____

_____

_____

Labeling
For each of the mercury-free thermometers shown below, write the temperature reading to the nearest tenth degree.

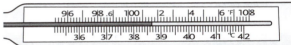

3. _____

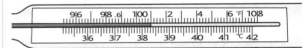

4. _____

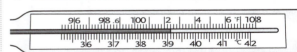

5. _____

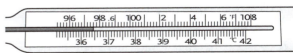

6. _____

Multiple Choice

7. Which of the following is the normal temperature range for the oral method?
   (A) 90.6 - 94.6 degrees F
   (B) 93.6 - 97.9 degrees F
   (C) 98.6 - 100.6 degrees F
   (D) 97.6 - 99.6 degrees F

8. Which of the following thermometers is used to take a temperature in the ear?
   (A) Oral thermometer
   (B) Rectal thermometer
   (C) Axillary thermometer
   (D) Tympanic thermometer

9. Which of the following temperature sites is another word for the armpit area?
   (A) Oral
   (B) Rectal
   (C) Axillary
   (D) Tympanic

10. Which temperature site is considered to be the most accurate?
    (A) Oral
    (B) Rectal
    (C) Axillary
    (D) Tympanic

11. Why are mercury-free thermometers considered safer than the mercury thermometers?
    (A) They do not contain mercury, which is a dangerous and toxic substance.
    (B) They are much smaller than mercury thermometers.
    (C) They are read differently than mercury thermometers.
    (D) They are less expensive than mercury thermometers.

12. How long do digital thermometers take to display a person's temperature?
    (A) 2 to 60 seconds
    (B) 1 to 2 minutes
    (C) 3 minutes
    (D) Less than 1 second

13. How many times are disposable thermometers used before being discarded?
    (A) Once
    (B) Twice
    (C) Three times
    (D) Five times

3. List guidelines for taking pulse and respirations

Multiple Choice

1. Where is the apical pulse located?
   (A) Underneath a person's chin
   (B) On the inside of the wrist
   (C) On the inside of the elbow
   (D) On the left side of the chest, just below the nipple

2. What is the most common site for monitoring the pulse?
   (A) Apical pulse
   (B) Femoral pulse
   (C) Pedal pulse
   (D) Radial pulse

3. For adults, the normal pulse rate is
   (A) 40–60 beats per minute
   (B) 60–100 beats per minute
   (C) 90–120 beats per minute
   (D) 20–40 beats per minute

4. Which of the following is an instrument that can listen to sounds within the body?
   (A) Reflex hammer
   (B) Scalpel
   (C) Stethoscope
   (D) Microscope

5. Breathing air into the lungs is also called
   (A) Inspiration
   (B) Expiration
   (C) Rhythm
   (D) Pulse

6. Exhaling air out of the lungs is also called
   (A) Inspiration
   (B) Expiration
   (C) Rhythm
   (D) Pulse

7. The normal respiration rate for adults ranges from
   (A) 5 to 10 breaths per minute
   (B) 12 to 20 breaths per minute
   (C) 25 to 32 breaths per minute
   (D) 7 to 11 breaths per minute

8. Why is it important to observe respirations without letting residents know that is what you are doing?
   (A) People may breathe more quickly if they know they are being observed.
   (B) People will hold their breath if they know what you want to measure.
   (C) It is illegal to gather information on respirations if you admit what you are doing beforehand.
   (D) Observing respirations is a painful process for most people.

4. Explain guidelines for taking blood pressure

Matching
For each of the following, write the letter of the correct definition from the list.

1. _____ 100–119 mmHg

2. _____ 60–79 mmHg

3. _____ diastolic phase

4. _____ hypertension

5. _____ hypotension

6. _____ mmHg

7. _____ sphygmomanometer

8. _____ systolic phase

(A) Blood pressure in the arteries when the heart is at work

(B) Low blood pressure

(C) Blood pressure in the arteries when the heart is at rest

(D) High blood pressure

(E) Blood pressure cuff

(F) Normal range for diastolic blood pressure

(G) Measuring unit used for blood pressure

(H) Normal range for systolic blood pressure

Short Answer

9. List five factors that can raise blood pressure.

_____

_____

_____

_____

_____

_____

_____

5. Describe guidelines for pain management

Short Answer

1. What questions should you ask to get the most accurate information if a resident complains of pain?

_____

_____

_____

_____

_____

_____

_____

2. Name ten signs and symptoms of pain that should be reported to the nurse.

_____

_____

_____

_____

_____

_____

_____

_____

_____

_____

_____

_____

Name: _____

3. List five measures that can help reduce a resident's pain.

_____

_____

_____

_____

_____

_____

_____

_____

_____

_____

6. Explain the benefits of warm and cold applications

Short Answer

Read each application or benefit below and decide if they relate to warm applications, cold applications, or both. Write "W" for warm (or heat), "C" for cold, or "B" for both.

1. ____ Prevents swelling

2. ____ Relieves muscular tension

3. ____ Aquamatic K-pad

4. ____ Tub baths

5. ____ Elevates temperature in tissues

6. ____ Relieves pain

7. ____ Increases blood flow

8. ____ Helps bring more oxygen and nutrients to tissues for healing

9. ____ Soaks

10. ____ Helps stop bleeding

11. ____ Brings down fever

12. ____ Compresses

13. ____ Sitz baths

True or False

14. ____ Moisture reduces the effect of heat and cold.

15. ____ Moist applications are less likely to cause injury than dry applications.

16. ____ Redness, pain, blisters, or numbness are signs that an application may be causing tissue damage.

17. ____ A sitz bath is a warm soak of the perineal area.

18. ____ Circulation is decreased by a sitz bath.

19. ____ Sitz baths may stimulate voiding.

20. ____ Residents may feel weak or dizzy after a sitz bath.

7. Explain how to apply non-sterile dressings and discuss sterile dressings

Fill in the Blank

1. Sterile dressings cover

   _____

   or _____

   wounds.

2. A _____

   changes sterile dressings.

3. Non-sterile dressings are applied to dry,

   _____

   wounds that have less chance of

   _____.

4. Nursing assistants may

   _____

   with non-sterile dressing changes.

Short Answer

5. What may nursing assistants be asked to do with regard to sterile dressings?

   _____

   _____

   _____

   _____

   _____

6. What are the supplies that may be needed for a sterile dressing change?

_____

_____

_____

_____

_____

7. What should nursing assistants observe and report about the wound site during sterile dressing changes?

_____

_____

_____

_____

_____

8. Discuss guidelines for non-sterile bandages

Multiple Choice

1. Elastic bandages are also known as
   (A) Non-sterile bandages
   (B) Plastic bandages
   (C) Liquid bandages
   (D) Aseptic bandages

2. One purpose of elastic bandages is to
   (A) Elevate a cast
   (B) Hold a dressing in place
   (C) Cover pressure sores
   (D) Help with ambulation

3. Apply elastic bandages snugly enough to control _____ and prevent movement of _____.
   (A) Temperature, the resident
   (B) Bleeding, dressings
   (C) Elevation, dressings
   (D) Movement, temperature

4. How soon should an NA check on a resident after applying a bandage?
   (A) 60 minutes
   (B) The next day
   (C) 5 hours
   (D) 15 minutes

9. List care guidelines for a resident who is on an IV

Multiple Choice

1. IVs allow direct access to
   (A) The heart
   (B) The lungs
   (C) The bloodstream
   (D) The muscles

2. What is the NA's responsibility for IV care?
   (A) Inserting IV lines
   (B) Removing IV lines
   (C) Care of the IV site
   (D) Documenting and reporting observations of changes or problems

Short Answer

3. List eight items that should be observed and reported about IVs.

_____

_____

_____

_____

_____

_____

_____

_____

_____

_____

_____

_____

10. Discuss oxygen therapy and explain related care guidelines

Multiple Choice

1. Which of the following is a box-like device that changes air in the room into air with more oxygen?
   (A) Oxygen cannula
   (B) Oxygen face mask
   (C) Oxygen concentrator
   (D) Oxygen prongs

2. When is it acceptable for you stop, adjust, or administer a resident's oxygen?
   (A) Whenever the resident requests that you do so
   (B) Every three days
   (C) Once per shift
   (D) Never

3. What is a cannula used for?
   (A) To provide nitrogen to the resident
   (B) To lock a wheelchair in place
   (C) To provide concentrated oxygen through a resident's nose
   (D) To secure a face mask to a resident who only occasionally needs oxygen

4. Liquid oxygen can cause which of the following?
   (A) Frostbite
   (B) Drug abuse or misuse
   (C) Digestive problems
   (D) Sterile water

5. What kind of water is used in humidifying bottles for oxygen concentrators?
   (A) Sparkling water
   (B) Purified water from natural springs
   (C) Sterile water
   (D) Tap water

6. What is the purpose of a humidifier?
   (A) To put only warm moisture in the air
   (B) To remove moisture from the air
   (C) To put warm or cool moisture in the air
   (D) To clean the air without adding moisture

15

Nutrition and Hydration

1. Describe the importance of good nutrition

Fill in the Blank

1. _____ is how the body uses food to maintain health.

2. Bodies need a balanced

   _____

   with nutrients and plenty of

   _____.

3. Good nutrition helps the body grow new

   _____ and

   have _____.

4. For the ill or elderly, a balanced diet can help prevent _____.

5. A good diet promotes

   _____

   and helps the body cope with

   _____.

2. List the six basic nutrients and explain the USDA's MyPyramid

Short Answer
Read the following sentences and mark which of the six basic nutrients they are describing. Use a "P" for proteins, "C" for carbohydrates, "F" for fats, "V" for vitamins, "M" for minerals, and "W" for water.

1. _____ Good sources of these are fish, meat, dried beans, soy products, and cheese.

2. _____ Without this, a person can only live a few days.

3. _____ These help the body store energy and provide insulation.

4. _____ These add flavor to food and help to absorb certain vitamins.

5. _____ They are essential for tissue growth and repair.

6. _____ Examples of these are butter, oil, and salad dressing.

7. _____ The body cannot make most of these; they can only be obtained from food.

8. _____ These provide fiber.

9. _____ Examples of these include bread, cereal, and potatoes.

10. _____ This is the most essential nutrient for life.

11. _____ These can be classified as monounsaturated, polyunsaturated, and saturated.

12. _____ Through perspiration, this helps to maintain body temperature.

13. _____ These can be fat-soluble or water-soluble.

14. _____ One-half to two-thirds of our body weight is this.

15. _____ Iron and calcium are examples of these.

Labeling
Looking at the USDA's MyPyramid below, fill in the seven areas.

16. _____

17. _____

18. _____

19. _____

20. _____

Name: _____

21. _____

22. _____

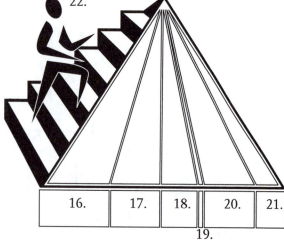

Short Answer

23. Describe your diet during the last 24 hours and break it down into food groups and servings.

_____

_____

_____

_____

_____

_____

_____

_____

_____

_____

_____

_____

Multiple Choice

24. MyPyramid is made up of six colored bands, which represent
(A) Different types of grains
(B) Different food groups
(C) Red meat and pork
(D) Ideal weights

25. What types of food should form the "base" of a healthy diet?
(A) Foods that are nutrient-dense and low in fat
(B) Foods that are high in fat and sugar
(C) Meats and dairy products
(D) Oils containing fatty acids

26. Most of your fruit choices should be
(A) Frozen fruit
(B) Smoothies
(C) Cut-up or whole fruit
(D) Fruit juice

27. How much vigorous activity does the USDA recommend you get per day?
(A) 60 minutes
(B) 20 minutes
(C) 10 minutes
(D) 30 minutes

28. Wheat, rice, oats, cornmeal, and barley are examples of which food group?
(A) Vegetables
(B) Fruits
(C) Grains
(D) Meat and beans

3. Identify nutritional problems of the elderly or ill

Short Answer

1. What can unintended weight loss lead to?

_____

_____

_____

_____

2. List five things to observe and report to the nurse about unintended weight loss.

_____

_____

_____

_____

_____

Name: _____

Word Search
Complete each of the following sentences and find your answers in the word search.

3. Encourage residents to
    _____.

4. Provide _____
    before and after meals.

5. Honor _____
    likes and dislikes.

6. Offer many different kinds of foods and
    _____.

7. Allow enough _____
    to finish eating.

8. Notify the nurse if a resident has trouble
    using _____.

9. Position residents sitting
    _____ for feeding.

10. If resident has had a loss of
    _____,
    ask about it.

11. Record meal/snack
    _____.

```
e u a x w e r a c l a r o u
e k j i l n s t u m b b p s
j e a e j e t s w y e r y e
l r t t p s f l v v i g z c
q c x i n z k n e g p a p d
l j o f t i g r h p y e p o
i v p i c e a t u e s v b h
b w m v m g p c m d v a a x
j n o u e j z p l u j q l m
d o q s w f z l a o b w m w
t a t d b n t o x m e c l p
c a o o u d x g e k d m z n
e o w i x v a g c c d c i u
f u t e n s i l s i i w c t
```

Short Answer

12. What is a nasogastric tube?

_____

_____

_____

_____

13. What is a gastrostomy?

_____

_____

_____

_____

14. What is total parenteral nutrition (TPN)?

_____

_____

_____

_____

4. Describe factors that influence food preferences

Short Answer

1. Briefly describe some of the foods you ate while growing up. Were there any special dishes that your family made that were related to your culture, religion, or region?

_____

_____

_____

_____

_____

_____

_____

_____

2. What rights do residents have with regard to food choices?

_____

_____

_____

_____

_____

_____

5. Explain the role of the dietary department

Short Answer

1. What is the role of the dietary department?

_____

_____

_____

_____

_____

2. When planning meals, what factors does the dietary department consider?

_____

_____

_____

_____

_____

3. What information is contained on diet cards?

_____

_____

_____

_____

6. Explain special diets

Matching
Read the following sentences and identify what special diet each is describing. Choose from the diets listed below.

1. _____ To prevent further heart or kidney damage, physicians may restrict a resident's fluid intake on this diet.

2. _____ This diet consists of foods that are in a liquid state at body temperature and are usually ordered as "clear" or "full."

3. _____ This diet consists of soft or chopped foods that are easy to chew and swallow, and is ordered for residents who have trouble chewing and swallowing due to dental problems or other medical conditions.

4. _____ In addition to restricted intake of fluids and sodium, people who have kidney disease may also be on this diet.

5. _____ This diet decreases the amount of fiber, whole grains, raw fruits and vegetables, and seeds consumed.

6. _____ Foods high in this mineral that may be increased in this diet include bananas, grapefruit, oranges, orange juice, prune juice, prunes, sweet potatoes, and winter squash.

7. _____ People at risk for heart attacks and heart disease may be placed on these. This diet includes limiting fatty meats, egg yolks, and fried foods.

8. _____ Calories and carbohydrates must be carefully regulated in this diet. The types of foods and the amounts are determined by the person's nutritional and energy requirements.

9. _____ Salt is restricted in this diet. Other high-sodium foods, such as ham, nuts, pickles, and canned soups, will be limited.

10. _____ This diet is used for losing weight or preventing additional weight gain.

11. _____ The food used in this diet has been blended or ground into a thick paste

of baby-food consistency; it is often used for people who have trouble chewing and/or swallowing more tex-tured foods.

12. _____ This diet increases the intake of fiber and whole grains, such as whole grain cereals, bread, and raw fruits and vegetables, to help prevent problems like constipation.

13. _____ This diet avoids foods that produce or increase levels of acid in the stomach, such as alcohol and beverages containing caffeine.

(A) Low-sodium diet

(B) Fluid-restricted diet

(C) Low-protein diet

(D) Low-fat/low-cholesterol diet

(E) Modified calorie diet

(F) Bland diet

(G) Dietary management of diabetes

(H) Soft diet and mechanical soft diet

(I) Pureed diet

(J) High-potassium diet

(K) Low-residue diet

(L) High-residue diet

(M) Liquid diet

7. Explain thickened liquids and identify three basic thickened consistencies

True or False

1. _____ Thickened liquids are usually ordered for residents with urinary problems.

2. _____ Thickening improves the ability to control fluids in the mouth and throat.

3. _____ A speech language pathologist will evaluate the resident to determine the thickness that the resident requires.

4. _____ Beverages will always arrive pre-thick-ened from the dietary department.

5. _____ A resident who must have thickened liquids may also drink water.

6. _____ Liquids that are nectar thick must be consumed with a spoon.

7. _____ A spoon should stand up straight in a glass of liquid that is pudding thick.

8. Describe how to make dining enjoyable for residents

Crossword
Fill in the blanks below and use your answers to complete the crossword puzzle.

Across

1. Give more _____ when requested.

5. Mealtime is not only the time for getting proper nourishment, but it is also a time for _____, which has a positive effect on eating.

7. Help residents _____ hands before eating.

Down

2. Encourage the use of _____, glasses, and hearing aids.

3. Give the resident the proper _____ devices to use for eating, if needed.

4. Proper position for eating is _____, which helps prevent swallowing problems.

6. Check the environment. The temperature should be comfortable. Keep noise level _____.

Name: _____

_____

_____

Scenarios

Read each scenario below and make suggestions for making mealtime more enjoyable for the resident.

8. Mrs. Peterson is a visually impaired resident. At mealtimes, she cannot see her food very well and complains that everything looks the same.

    _____

    _____

    _____

    _____

9. Mr. Leisering comes to dinner in his pajamas. His hair has not been brushed and he is wearing slippers instead of shoes.

    _____

    _____

    _____

    _____

10. Ms. Lopez does not speak very much English, and she has not met any of the other Spanish-speaking residents. She comes to meals wrapped in a large sweater and jumps every time she hears trays clattering or when someone raises his voice.

    _____

    _____

    _____

    _____

    _____

11. Mr. Gaines has dentures, but he says that they give him pain so he often does not wear them while eating. It takes him a long time to finish his meals, and he has to concentrate so hard on chewing his food that he does not seem interested in conversation with anyone around him.

    _____

    _____

    _____

9. Explain how to serve meal trays and assist with eating

True or False

1. _____ You should take your time serving residents their dinner so that they will not feel rushed.

2. _____ All residents sitting together at one table should be served at the same time so that they may eat together.

3. _____ It is important to identify each resident before serving meal trays.

4. _____ You should do as much as possible for each resident so the meal can proceed quickly.

5. _____ If a resident needs his food cut, it should be done before the food is brought to the table.

6. _____ You should open milk and juice cartons, straws, and condiment packets for residents.

7. _____ Straws are helpful for residents with swallowing problems.

8. _____ Pureed food should not be seasoned.

9. _____ Remain silent while helping a resident eat.

10. _____ If food is too hot, blow on it for a few minutes until it is cool enough for the resident to eat it.

11. _____ Residents should be sitting upright at a 90-degree angle for eating.

12. _____ If a resident wants to eat his dessert first, tell him "no" and explain that it is unhealthy and that you are only doing what is best for him.

13. _____ Alternating cold and hot foods or bland foods and sweets can help increase appetite.

14. _____ If a resident does not want to wear a clothing protector, tell her that she needs to or else her clothes will be soiled and she will have to change.

Scenarios

Read each scenario below and describe how each
NA can improve her technique of assisting at meals.

15. Mrs. Rains, a Catholic resident, asks Carol
    to join her in a small prayer before she eats.
    Carol declines, explaining that she does
    not believe in God and thinks that prayer is
    pointless.

    _____

    _____

    _____

    _____

    _____

16. Tracy had a fight with her husband this
    morning and is in a very bad mood. Mrs.
    Foster, a friendly resident, tries to make con-
    versation with Tracy as she is handing out
    meal trays. "I don't have time to talk right
    now," Tracy snaps at her. "Can't you see how
    much I have to do?"

    _____

    _____

    _____

    _____

    _____

17. Mr. Parks, a resident with arthritis, can usu-
    ally feed himself, but today his hands are
    hurting him so much that he cannot hold
    the utensils or even his napkin. Carol helps
    him eat while joking loudly with the other
    residents that he must be feeling like royalty
    having someone wait on him hand and foot.

    _____

    _____

    _____

    _____

18. Mr. Correll is recovering from pneumonia.
    Pam serves his meal and then watches for
    a few moments to see if he needs any help.
    When she determines that he can feed him-
    self, she goes on to help another resident.
    After she leaves, Mr. Correll starts to feel
    weak and begins having trouble lifting the
    utensils to his mouth. He waits for 15 min-
    utes for someone to come back to help him
    finish his meal.

    _____

    _____

    _____

    _____

    _____

    _____

19. While handing out meal trays, Pam notices
    that Mr. Gray's diet card indicates a low-
    sodium diet but his meal tray contains a
    meal for residents with no restrictions. She
    assumes his diet must have changed and
    gives him the tray.

    _____

    _____

    _____

    _____

    _____

20. Mrs. Palmer has Parkinson's disease. She
    can feed herself, but she does so very slowly,
    as her hands are sometimes shaky. Tracy
    cuts Mrs. Palmer's food and feeds it to her
    so that it will not take her so long to finish.

    _____

    _____

    _____

    _____

    _____

10. Describe how to assist residents with special needs

Fill in the Blank.

1. Use _____ devices such as utensils with built-up handle grips, plate guards, and drinking cups when necessary.

2. For visually-impaired residents, use the face of an imaginary

   _____

   to explain the position of what is in front of them.

3. For residents who have had a stroke, place food in the unaffected, or

   _____,

   side of the mouth.

4. Residents with Parkinson's disease may need help if

   _____

   or shaking make it difficult for them to eat.

5. The hand-over-hand approach is an example of a physical

   _____

   that can help promote independence.

6. Verbal cues must be short and

   _____

   and prompt the resident to do something.

7. If a resident has poor sitting balance, seat him or her in a regular dining room chair with armrests, rather than in a

   _____.

   Put the resident in the proper position in the chair, which means hips at a

   _____ -

   degree angle, knees flexed, and feet and arms fully supported.

8. If the resident bites down on utensils, ask him to

   _____

   his mouth.

9. If the resident pockets food in his cheeks, ask him to chew and

   _____

   the food.

11. Define "dysphagia" and identify signs and symptoms of swallowing problems

Short Answer

1. What should you do if you see signs of dysphagia in a resident?

   _____

   _____

   _____

   _____

2. List 14 signs and symptoms of dysphagia that must be reported.

   _____

   _____

   _____

   _____

   _____

   _____

   _____

   _____

   _____

   _____

   _____

   _____

   _____

   _____

12. Explain intake and output (I&O)

True or False

1. ____ Fluids come in the form of liquids you drink as well as semi-liquid foods such as soup or gelatin.

2. ____ The fluid a person consumes is called intake or input.

3. ____ All of the body's fluid output is in the form of urine.

4. ____ Fluid balance is taking in and eliminating the same amounts of fluid.

5. ____ Most people need to consciously monitor their fluid balance.

Conversions

6. A healthy person generally needs to take in about 64 to 96 ounces (oz.) of fluid each day. How many milliliters (mL) is this?

_____ to

_____ mL. How many

cups is this? _____

cups.

7. Mrs. Hedman drinks half of a glass of orange juice. You know that the glass holds about 1 cup of liquid. How many mL of orange juice did Mrs. Hedman drink?

_____

8. Mr. Ramirez just ate some chocolate pudding from a 6-oz. container. You measure the leftover pudding, which is about 35 mL. How many mL of pudding did Mr. Ramirez eat? _____

9. Miss Sumiko has a bowl of soup for lunch. The soup bowl holds about 1 ½ cups of liquid.

Convert this to mL. _____.
Miss Sumiko finishes most of her soup, but there is about 25 mL left. How many mL of soup did Miss Sumiko eat?

_____

10. After his lunch, Mr. Lake selected orange-flavored gelatin for dessert. He was given one cup of gelatin, but he only ate about ¼ of it. How many mL of gelatin did he consume?

_____

How many mL were left over?

_____

11. Mr. Weiss indicates that he needs to use the bathroom. He uses a urinal to help with measurement of his I&O. According to the graduate, Mr. Lake outputs two cups of urine. How many mL is this?

_____

13. Identify ways to assist residents in maintaining fluid balance

True or False

1. _____ Drinking 12 ounces of water per day is the recommended amount for most people.

2. _____ Force fluids means to restrict the amount of fluids consumed.

3. _____ Fluid overload occurs when the body is unable to handle the amount of fluid consumed.

4. _____ If a resident has an order for "NPO," this means he can drink water but nothing else.

5. _____ The sense of thirst lessens as a person ages.

6. _____ People can become dehydrated by vomiting too much.

7. _____ A symptom of fluid overload is edema of the extremities.

8. _____ In order to prevent dehydration, offer fresh fluids often.

9. _____ A symptom of dehydration is dark urine.

10. _____ It is a good idea for residents with swallowing problems to suck on ice chips.

11. _____ Make sure that the water pitcher and cup are near enough and light enough for the resident to lift.

16

Urinary Elimination

1. List qualities of urine and identify signs and symptoms about urine to report

Multiple Choice

1. Urine is composed of water and
   (A) Dye
   (B) Blood
   (C) Waste products
   (D) Plasma

2. Generally, adults should produce about
   _____ mL of urine per day.
   (A) 2400 to 2800
   (B) 25 to 50
   (C) 400 to 700
   (D) 1200 to 1500

3. How should urine normally appear?
   (A) Pale yellow or amber
   (B) Rust-colored
   (C) Red
   (D) Cloudy

Labeling
Mark an "X" next to each of the following items that is a sign or symptom that should be reported to the nurse.

4. ____ Urinary incontinence

5. ____ Urine has faint smell

6. ____ Urine is pale yellow in color

7. ____ Blood, pus, mucus, or discharge in urine

8. ____ Urine is transparent

9. ____ Painful urination

10. ____ Protein or glucose in urine

11. ____ Cloudy urine

12. ____ Urine has fruity smell

13. ____ Dark or rust-colored urine

14. ____ Urine has strong smell

2. List factors affecting urination and demonstrate how to assist with elimination

True or False

1. ____ As a person ages, the bladder is not able to hold the same amount of urine.

2. ____ Diuretics are medications that can cause frequent urination.

3. ____ When assisting with perineal care, make sure to wipe from back to front.

4. ____ A healthy person needs to take in from 64 to 96 ounces of fluid each day.

5. ____ To promote privacy during urination, close the bathroom door or pull the privacy curtain and close the door.

6. ____ As a person ages, he or she becomes more thirsty.

7. ____ Alcohol and caffeine increase urine output.

8. ____ Diabetes can affect urination.

Multiple Choice

9. A fracture pan is used for voiding for
   (A) Any resident who cannot get out of bed
   (B) Residents who cannot raise their hips
   (C) Residents who have problems with incontinence
   (D) Residents who have difficulty urinating

10. Men will generally use a _____ for urination when they cannot get out of bed.
(A) Urinal
(B) Fracture pan
(C) Toilet
(D) Portable commode

11. Residents who can get out of bed but cannot walk to the bathroom may use a
(A) Toilet
(B) Urinal
(C) Portable commode
(D) Indwelling catheter

12. When disposing of wastes, you should
(A) Always wear gloves
(B) Leave the container on the overbed table
(C) Dispose of them outside
(D) Ask the resident to take care of his or her own waste

3. Describe common diseases and disorders of the urinary system

True or False

1. _____ Cystitis is more common in men than it is in women.

2. _____ Urine irritates the skin and must be completely cleaned off.

3. _____ Functional incontinence is caused by overflow of the bladder.

4. _____ Calculi, or kidney stones, form when urine crystallizes in the kidneys.

5. _____ Kidney dialysis is used for cleaning mucus from the lungs.

6. _____ When a person has a UTI she may experience a painful burning sensation during urination and the frequent feeling of needing to urinate.

7. _____ To avoid infection, women should wipe the perineal area from front to back after elimination.

8. _____ Kidney stones can be the result of a vitamin deficiency or mineral imbalance.

9. _____ Nephritis may cause rusty-colored urine and a decrease in urine output.

10. _____ Excessive salt in the diet can cause damage to the kidneys.

11. _____ Incontinence is a normal part of aging.

12. _____ Incontinence can occur if a resident is bedbound, ill, elderly, paralyzed, or injured.

13. _____ Stress incontinence is involuntary voiding due to an abrupt urge.

14. _____ It is disrespectful to refer to incontinence briefs as "diapers."

4. Describe guidelines for urinary catheter care

Matching
Use each letter only once.

1. ____ Urinary catheter that has an attachment that fits onto the penis

2. ____ Urinary catheter that is removed immediately after urine is drained

3. ____ Thin tube used to drain urine from the bladder

4. ____ Urinary catheter that stays inside the bladder for a period of time

5. ____ Thin tube inserted into the body that is used to drain or inject fluids

(A) Indwelling catheter

(B) Condom catheter

(C) Straight catheter

(D) Catheter

(E) Urinary catheter

Short Answer

6. List three guidelines to follow when working around residents with catheters.

_____

_____

_____

_____

_____

_____

_____

7. List six things to report to the nurse about a resident's catheter.

_____

_____

_____

_____

_____

_____

5. Identify types of urine specimens that are collected

Letters may be used more than once.

1. ____ Collection container put into toilet to collect samples

2. ____ Tests for bacteria in urine

3. ____ Also called "mid-stream" specimen

4. ____ A sample that is used for analysis in order to try to make a diagnosis

5. ____ Tests for certain chemicals and hormones

6. ____ Collects all urine voided in 24 hours

7. ____ Urine sample collected any time resident voids

8. ____ Excludes first and last urine from sample

(A) 24-hour urine specimen

(B) Clean catch specimen

(C) Hat

(D) Routine urine specimen

(E) Specimen

6. Explain types of tests performed on urine

Multiple Choice

1. A reagent strip
    (A) Tests for food in urine
    (B) Tests for pH level in urine
    (C) Tests for illegal drugs in urine
    (D) Tests for fat in urine

2. The presence of glucose or ketones in urine may be a sign of
    (A) High blood pressure
    (B) Thyroid disorder
    (C) Anemia
    (D) Diabetes

3. "Occult" blood in urine is
    (A) A normal change of aging
    (B) Easy to see
    (C) Hidden
    (D) Anemic

4. A urine specific gravity test
    (A) Checks oxygen levels in the blood
    (B) Shows how urine compares to stool
    (C) Determines amount of white blood cells
    (D) Shows how urine compares to water

5. A double-voided urine specimen may be used to test for
    (A) Glucose
    (B) Sweat
    (C) Sputum
    (D) Immunity

7. Explain guidelines for assisting with bladder retraining

Scenarios

Ms. Potter has been staying at the Cool River Retirement Center for several months while she recovers from a broken hip. Her recovery is proceeding well, but she has had a problem with urinary incontinence since her injury. Her doctor tells the nurses and NAs on Ms. Potter's unit to assist her with bladder retraining.

Below are examples of how three of the NAs help Ms. Potter with retraining. Read each one and state what the NA is doing well and/or what he or she should do differently.

1. Hannah, a new nursing assistant, wants to be very professional about the episodes of incontinence. While she is cleaning the bed, she remains very upbeat and friendly and does not mention the incontinence unless Ms. Potter brings it up.

_____

_____

_____

_____

_____

_____

_____

2. Greta senses Ms. Potter's acute embarrassment and it makes her nervous. Whenever she has to assist Ms. Potter, she speaks very little and does not make eye contact with her. She tries to finish her work as quickly as possible to limit Ms. Potter's discomfort.

_____

_____

_____

_____

_____

3. Pete has been very encouraging and positive with Ms. Potter. He has charted her bathroom schedule. He makes sure to be available to help her around the usual times that she needs to go to the bathroom. He responds to her call light quickly and compliments Ms. Potter on her retraining efforts.

_____

_____

_____

_____

_____

_____

_____

_____

17

Bowel Elimination

1. List qualities of stools and identify signs and symptoms to report about stool

True or False

1. ____ Defecation is the process of passing feces from the large intestine out of the body.

2. ____ Everyone should have the same number of bowel movements per day.

3. ____ Normal stool is watery and loose.

4. ____ Certain foods can change the color of stool.

5. ____ Stool that is whitish, black, or red should be reported to the nurse.

6. ____ Constipation is normal and does not need to be reported to the nurse.

7. ____ Fecal incontinence is normal for people over age 65 and should not be reported.

2. List factors affecting bowel elimination

Multiple Choice

1. Peristalsis is
   (A) Constipation
   (B) Contractions that move food through the GI system
   (C) Pain that can occur during elimination
   (D) Fecal or anal incontinence

2. Foods that are high in animal fats and refined sugar but low in fiber can
   (A) Improve bowel elimination
   (B) Cause constipation
   (C) Cause anal leakage
   (D) Cause weight loss

3. Normal bowel elimination is aided by
   (A) Proper fluid intake
   (B) Eating only red meat
   (C) Eating dairy products, such as cheese
   (D) All-liquid diets

4. The best position for bowel elimination is
   (A) Lying supine on the back
   (B) Lying prone on the abdomen
   (C) Reclining 45 degrees
   (D) Squatting and leaning forward

5. Bowel elimination usually occurs
   (A) Morning, noon, and night
   (B) After meals
   (C) In the supine position
   (D) During physical activity

3. Describe common diseases and disorders of the gastrointestinal system

Crossword

Across

2. GERD occurs when stomach contents back up into the
   _____.

5. _____
   are enlarged veins in the rectum that cause itching and burning.

7. If heartburn occurs frequently and remains untreated, it can cause scarring or
   _____.

9. Ulcerative colitis is a chronic inflammatory disease of the large
   _____.

Name: _____

10. Raw sores in the stomach or small intestine are called

_____ .

13. Treatment of

_____

often includes increasing the amount of fiber eaten.

14. To prevent heartburn and GERD, provide an extra pillow to make the resident's body more

_____

during sleep.

Down

1. Surgical treatment of ulcerative colitis may include a

_____ .

3. Constipation occurs when the feces move too slowly through the intestine as the result of decreased

_____

intake and poor diet.

4. Cancer of the gastrointestinal tract is

_____

cancer.

6. Heartburn is a result of a weakening of the

_____

muscle that joins the esophagus and the stomach.

8. A diet of bananas, rice, apples, and tea/toast is called the

_____

diet.

11. Residents with peptic ulcers should avoid

_____

and drinking alcohol.

12. _____

is the frequent elimination of liquid or semi-liquid feces.

4. Discuss how enemas are given

Short Answer

1. Why are enemas given?

_____

_____

_____

_____

_____

2. What position must a resident be in when getting an enema?

_____

_____

_____

3. If the resident has pain or if you feel resistance while giving an enema, what should you do?

_____

_____

_____

4. How can the resident's legal rights be protected while giving an enema?

_____

_____

_____

_____

_____

5. Demonstrate how to collect a stool specimen

True or False

1. _____ Stool is often tested for blood, pathogens, or worms.

2. _____ An ova and parasites test is used to detect occult blood in stool.

3. _____ Ova and parasites tests must be done while the stool is still warm.

4. _____ Urine or paper can ruin a stool sample.

6. Explain occult blood testing

Fill in the Blank

1. Hidden blood in stool is called

_____

blood.

2. Blood in stool may be a sign of a serious problem, such as

_____

or other illnesses.

3. One test for blood in stool is called the

_____

test.

7. Define the term "ostomy" and list care guidelines

True or False

1. _____ An ostomy is an operation to create an opening from an area inside the body to the outside.

2. _____ A stoma is an artificial opening in the abdomen through which stool is eliminated.

3. _____ In a colostomy, the stool will generally be semi-solid.

4. _____ In an ileostomy, the stool will generally be solid.

Short Answer

5. Why do you think a resident with an ostomy might feel embarrassed about it?

_____

_____

_____

_____

Multiple Choice

6. How often should an ostomy bag be emptied and cleaned or replaced?
   (A) Once a day
   (B) Every hour
   (C) Whenever a stool is eliminated
   (D) Before a resident wakes up

7. What could cause a food blockage in a resident who has an ileostomy?
   (A) Too much liquid in the resident's diet
   (B) A large amount of high-fiber food in the resident's diet
   (C) Skin irritation
   (D) Cold compresses

8. Explain guidelines for assisting with bowel retraining

Word Search

1. Residents who have had a disruption in their bowel _____ may need help to restore normal

_____.

Name: _____

2. Wear _____
   when handling body wastes.

3. Explain the training
   _____ to the resident.
   Keep a _____ of
   bowel habits.

4. Encourage plenty of
   _____

   and foods that are high in

   _____.

5. Provide _____
   in the bed and bathroom.

6. Help with _____
   care, which can prevent skin breakdown.

7. Discard clothing _____
   and _____
   briefs properly.

8. Praise _____
   and _____
   to control bowels.

9. Never show _____
   or _____
   toward an incontinent resident.

```
s  f  r  w  e  s  l  a  e  n  i  r  e  p
e  u  e  e  c  i  u  p  a  t  i  e  n  t
n  n  c  h  n  s  e  c  m  b  q  a  y  m
i  c  o  n  e  y  t  f  c  z  j  c  z  n
t  t  r  q  n  g  g  p  h  e  a  c  o  r
u  i  d  c  i  u  l  n  m  v  s  i  z  s
o  o  x  t  t  r  d  o  i  e  t  s  c  d
r  n  m  k  n  a  e  r  v  a  t  h  e  f
e  c  r  z  o  d  p  g  r  e  e  t  l  s
y  m  s  r  c  j  j  t  n  d  s  u  a  y
q  s  t  r  n  b  s  s  u  a  i  e  p  c
u  u  o  y  i  u  z  l  z  d  t  j  z  j
p  d  h  a  r  e  e  w  s  r  e  b  i  f
t  x  b  f  p  r  o  t  e  c  t  o  r  s
```

18

Common Chronic and Acute Conditions

1. Describe common diseases and disorders of the integumentary system

Matching
Use each letter only once.

1. _____ Caused by fungal imbalances; athlete's foot, vaginal yeast infections, and ringworm are examples

2. _____ Contagious skin condition caused by a tiny mite that burrows into the skin, where it lays eggs; this condition is spread through direct contact with an infected person

3. _____ A type of injury to the skin; classified as either open or closed

4. _____ Skin rash caused by the varicella-zoster virus (VZV), which is the same virus that causes chickenpox

5. _____ A general term that refers to an inflammation, or swelling, of the skin

6. _____ A skin condition that occurs due to build-up of fluid under the skin; commonly affects the lower legs and ankles

(A) Dermatitis

(B) Fungal infections

(C) Scabies

(D) Shingles

(E) Stasis dermatitis

(F) Wounds

2. Describe common diseases and disorders of the musculoskeletal system

Multiple Choice

Arthritis

1. Arthritis is a general term referring to _____ of the joints.
   (A) Immobility
   (B) Swelling
   (C) Redness
   (D) Stiffness

2. Arthritis may be the result of
   (A) Improper infection prevention measures
   (B) Amputation
   (C) Autoimmune illness
   (D) Substance abuse

3. What happens with an autoimmune illness?
   (A) The circulatory system stops functioning.
   (B) The immune system attacks diseased tissue in the body.
   (C) The immune system attacks normal tissue in the body.
   (D) The chain of infection is broken.

4. Osteoarthritis is common in
   (A) The elderly
   (B) Infants
   (C) Teenagers
   (D) Nursing assistants

5. Pain and stiffness of osteoarthritis may increase with
   (A) Hot weather
   (B) Cold weather
   (C) Activity
   (D) Dehydration

6. Rheumatoid arthritis affects the _____ joints first.
   (A) Smaller
   (B) Larger
   (C) Elbow
   (D) There is no typical progression

7. Arthritis is generally treated with
   (A) Botox
   (B) Plastic surgery
   (C) Deep breathing exercises
   (D) Anti-inflammatory medications

Osteoporosis

True or False

8. ____ Osteoporosis causes bones to become brittle and break easily.

9. ____ Residents with osteoporosis must be moved very carefully.

10. ____ Osteoporosis is more common in women before menopause.

11. ____ Exercise and extra calcium can help prevent osteoporosis.

12. ____ There is no treatment for osteoporosis.

Fractures

Multiple Choice

13. When caring for a resident who has a cast, _____ the extremity that is in a cast to help stop swelling.
    (A) Lower
    (B) Double bandage
    (C) Elevate
    (D) Shake

14. Keep the cast _____ and clean at all times.
    (A) Dry
    (B) Wet
    (C) Hot
    (D) Pointed

15. A bone must be _____ to allow the fusion of fractured parts.
    (A) Lowered
    (B) Moved
    (C) Wet
    (D) Immobilized

16. Signs and symptoms of a fracture include
    (A) Heat
    (B) Cold
    (C) Swelling
    (D) Dryness

17. Fractures are broken bones and may be caused by
    (A) Eating too much fiber
    (B) Talking
    (C) Osteoporosis
    (D) Laughing

18. You can place a wet cast on _____ so that its shape is not altered as it dries.
    (A) A metal surface
    (B) Pillows
    (C) Concrete
    (D) A wood floor

19. When can a resident insert something inside the cast?
    (A) When skin itches
    (B) After the cast dries
    (C) When the cast is wet
    (D) Never

20. A fracture that has penetrated the skin and carries a high risk of infection is called a(n)
    (A) Open fracture
    (B) Hairline fracture
    (C) Closed fracture
    (D) Infectious fracture

Hip Fractures

True or False

21. ____ Most fractured hips require surgery.

22. ____ You should perform ROM exercises for a leg on the side of a hip replacement when you see that the resident is in pain.

23. ____ A hip fracture is not really a serious injury.

24. ____ Elderly people heal slowly.

25. ____ Nursing assistants may disconnect traction assembly if the resident requests it.

26. _____ A resident recovering from a hip replacement should not sit with his or her legs crossed. The hip cannot be bent more than 90 degrees.

27. _____ Dress a resident recovering from a hip replacement starting with the unaffected, or stronger, side first.

28. _____ A red or warm incision after hip replacement surgery must be reported to the nurse.

Multiple Choice

29. What is the main reason that hip fractures are more common in the elderly?
    (A) Bones weaken as people age.
    (B) Elderly people get too much exercise.
    (C) Elderly people are depressed.
    (D) Elderly people can bear more weight on their bones.

30. Which side should residents recovering from hip replacements dress first?
    (A) Affected side
    (B) It does not matter.
    (C) Unaffected side
    (D) Left side, no matter which side is affected

31. What does "PWB" stand for?
    (A) Previously weakened bones
    (B) Partial weight bearing
    (C) Patient's weight before
    (D) Patient wants baths

32. If you see "NWB" on a resident's care plan, the resident:
    (A) Can support 100 percent of his or her body weight on one leg
    (B) Can support some weight, but not all, on one or both legs
    (C) Is unable to support any weight on one or both legs
    (D) Can use stairs without assistance

Knee Replacement

True or False

33. _____ A knee replacement may be done to relieve pain or restore motion to the knee.

34. _____ The recovery time for a knee replacement is longer than for a hip replacement.

35. _____ Compression stockings are applied to the legs and hooked to a machine that inflates and deflates to act as the muscles normally would.

36. _____ Ankle pumps are simple exercises to promote circulation to the legs.

37. _____ Fluid intake should be restricted after a knee replacement.

Muscular Dystrophy (MD)

True or False

38. _____ Muscular dystrophy is an inherited disease that causes gradual wasting of the muscles.

39. _____ Most forms of MD become apparent in middle adulthood.

40. _____ Many forms of MD are very slow to progress.

41. _____ In the late stages of MD, many residents will need you to perform their activities of daily living (ADLs) for them.

Amputation

Short Answer

42. What is phantom sensation? Is it real or should it be ignored?

_____

_____

_____

_____

43. Are there any complementary or alternative health practices that you use? If so, which ones?

_____

_____

_____

_____

_____

_____

_____

_____

3. Describe common diseases and disorders of the nervous system

CVA or Stroke

True or False

1. _____ Residents with paralysis or loss of movement do not need physical therapy.

2. _____ Range of motion exercises strengthen muscles and keep joints mobile.

3. _____ Leg exercises help improve circulation.

4. _____ When helping with transfers or ambulation, stand on the resident's stronger side.

5. _____ Always use a gait belt for safety when helping with transfers or walking.

6. _____ Refer to the side that has been affected by stroke as the "bad" side so that residents will understand which side you are talking about.

7. _____ Gestures and nonverbal communication are important in communicating with the CVA resident.

8. _____ Residents who suffer confusion or memory loss due to a stroke may feel more secure if you keep a routine of care.

9. _____ Residents with a loss of sensation could easily burn or cut themselves.

10. _____ Pay close attention to changes in the skin of the CVA resident, and observe for skin breakdown.

11. _____ Let the resident do things for him- or herself whenever possible.

Scenarios

Read each of the following statements, and answer the questions.

12. Jody, a nursing assistant, is getting ready to help feed Mr. Elliot, who is recovering from a stroke. Mr. Elliot has difficulty communicating and also suffers from confusion. "Let's see," Jody says. "For lunch you have soup, a sandwich, and a salad. Now, what would you like to eat?" What is wrong with the way Jody is communicating with Mr. Elliot?

_____

_____

_____

_____

_____

13. Mr. Elliot's daughter visits during meal time and asks how her dad is doing. Jody says, "Mr. Elliot is having trouble today with his eating. Just look at him. He's spilled all over himself." What is wrong with what Jody has just said?

_____

_____

_____

_____

14. Jody notices that Mr. Elliot seems to be having trouble saying words clearly. He is beginning to get frustrated because he cannot tell Jody what he wants. Jody decides to ask only yes or no questions, so she tells Mr. Elliot, "If you find it too difficult to speak right now, why don't you try nodding your head for 'yes' and shaking your head for 'no.'" What is Jody doing right?

_____

_____

_____

_____

_____

Fill in the Blank

15. When assisting with a transfer for a resident with one-sided weakness, always lead with the _____ side.

16. Dress the _____ side first. This prevents unnecessary bending.

17. Undress the _____ side first.

18. _____ equipment can be used to help the resident dress himself.

19. When assisting a CVA resident to eat, place the food in the resident's _____.

20. Always place food in the _____ side of the mouth.

Parkinson's Disease

True or False

21. _____ Parkinson's disease is a progressive disease that causes a section of the brain to degenerate.

22. _____ Parkinson's disease causes a shuffling gait and a mask-like facial expression.

23. _____ Pill-rolling is moving the thumb and first finger together like rolling a pill.

24. _____ Residents with Parkinson's disease should be discouraged from performing any of their own care.

Multiple Sclerosis (MS)

Fill in the Blank

25. Multiple sclerosis causes the protective _____ for the nerves, spinal cord, and white matter of the brain to break down over time.

26. For a person with MS, nerves cannot send _____ to and from the brain in a normal way.

27. Symptoms of MS include _____ vision, fatigue, poor _____, and trouble _____.

28. MS can cause loss of function in the _____ and _____.

29. Offer _____ periods as necessary for residents with MS.

30. Give residents plenty of time to _____.

31. _____ can worsen the effects of MS.

32. Range of motion exercises may prevent _____ and strengthen _____.

Head and Spinal Cord Injuries

True or False

33. _____ Head and spinal cord injuries are often caused by accidents, war, or criminal violence.

34. _____ Residents with head injuries may have personality changes, seizures, or memory loss.

35. _____ The effects of a spinal cord injury depend on the location of the injury and the force of impact.

36. _____ The lower the injury on the spinal cord, the greater the loss of function will be.

37. _____ Quadriplegia is a loss of function of the lower body and legs.

38. _____ Rehabilitation is of little help for residents with spinal cord injuries.

39. _____ Residents with injuries will need emotional support as well as physical help.

40. _____ People with these injuries may not feel burns because of loss of sensation.

41. _____ Frequent skin care and position changes can help prevent pressure sores. Assist residents to change positions at least every two hours to prevent pressure sores.

42. _____ Residents with spinal cord injuries should drink very little fluids.

Epilepsy

Short Answer

43. What is the main goal of the caregiver during a seizure?

_____

_____

_____

_____

_____

44. Why should you not put anything in a person's mouth when he or she is having a seizure?

_____

_____

_____

_____

45. Why should you notice the time a seizure begins?

_____

_____

_____

_____

Vision Impairment

Matching
Use each letter only once.

46. _____ The ability to see objects that are nearby better than objects in the distance

47. _____ Condition that causes increased pressure in the eye and eventual blindness

48. _____ Condition that causes cloudiness of the lens of the eye, which can cause vision to be lost

49. _____ The ability to see objects in the distance better than objects nearby

(A) Glaucoma

(B) Nearsightedness

(C) Farsightedness

(D) Cataract

4. Describe common diseases and disorders of the cardiovascular system

Short Answer

Hypertension (HTN) or High Blood Pressure

1. What is the difference between hypertension and prehypertension?

_____

_____

_____

_____

_____

_____

2. What are three possible causes of hypertension?

_____

_____

_____

_____

3. Why is treatment of hypertension important?

_____

_____

_____

_____

Coronary Artery Disease (CAD)

True or False

4. _____ Coronary artery disease (CAD) occurs when the coronary arteries widen and increase blood flow.

5. _____ CAD lowers the supply of blood, oxygen, and nutrients to the heart and can lead to heart attack or stroke.

6. _____ Angina pectoris is chest pain, pressure, or discomfort caused by reduced oxygen to the heart.

7. _____ The heart needs more oxygen when the body is at rest.

8. _____ The pain of angina pectoris is usually described as pressure or tightness in the left side of the chest.

9. _____ A person suffering from angina pectoris may sweat, look pale, and have trouble breathing.

10. _____ If a person with CAD rests, it helps the blood flow return to normal.

11. _____ Nursing assistants can give residents nitroglycerin if needed.

12. _____ Residents with CAD may need to avoid heavy meals and intense exercise.

Myocardial Infarction (MI) or Heart Attack

Short Answer

13. List five guidelines for residents recovering from a myocardial infarction.

_____

_____

_____

_____

_____

_____

_____

Congestive Heart Failure (CHF)

Short Answer

14. List five signs and symptoms of congestive heart failure.

_____

_____

_____

_____

_____

_____

Word Search

Fill in the blanks below and find your answers in the word search.

15. CHF can be controlled with

_____.

16. Medications help remove excess

_____.

This means more trips to the

_____.

17. Limited _____

or _____

may be prescribed.

18. Residents may be

_____

at the same time every day.

19. Extra _____

may help residents who have trouble breathing.

20. A common side effect of CHF medication is

_____.

```
d c g l p q y y b r x s r e
x i n f v d n k a p d w b l
w i z l o b s m t b w o u p
d h r z i d j q h p u l q i
l e v b i v z a r e e l z d
g u h u b n c h o t j i i c
b s l g q t e d o h h p m f
a f c f i v c s m m j o r v
m d n v m e y t s e r d e b
q t i e i q w l h t c v x r
e t q t q g r f t l o g z h
y m e d i c a t i o n w v u
n o c g f h s g g o c s x n
o p v m z q z k h r g t x z
```

Peripheral Vascular Disease (PVD)

Multiple Choice

21. Peripheral vascular disease (PVD) is a condition in which the legs, feet, arms, or hands do not have enough
    (A) Flexibility
    (B) Exercise
    (C) Blood circulation
    (D) Fluids

22. PVD is caused by
    (A) Incontinence
    (B) Weakened heart muscle due to damage
    (C) Infection
    (D) Fatty deposits in blood vessels

23. When do anti-embolic hose need to be applied?
    (A) Before the resident gets out of bed
    (B) While the resident is walking around
    (C) Right after a shower or tub bath
    (D) During meal time

5. Describe common diseases and disorders of the respiratory system

Chronic Obstructive Pulmonary Disease (COPD)

Multiple Choice

1. Residents with COPD have difficulty with
   (A) Breathing
   (B) Urination
   (C) Losing weight
   (D) Vision

2. A constant fear of a person who has COPD is
   (A) Constipation
   (B) Incontinence
   (C) Not being able to breathe
   (D) Heart attack

3. A resident with COPD should be positioned
   (A) Lying flat on his back
   (B) Sitting upright
   (C) Lying on his stomach
   (D) Lying on his side

4. Your role in caring for a resident with COPD includes
   (A) Being calm and supportive
   (B) Adjusting oxygen levels
   (C) Making changes in the resident's diet
   (D) Doing everything for the resident as much as possible

5. Chronic bronchitis and emphysema are grouped under
   (A) Chronic obstructive pulmonary disease, or COPD
   (B) Muscular dystrophy, or MD
   (C) Hypertension, or HTN
   (D) Coronary artery disease, or CAD

Matching

6. ____ Highly contagious lung disease; symptoms include coughing, low-grade fever, shortness of breath, weight loss, and fatigue

7. ____ Results from a bacterial or viral infection of the nose, sinuses, and throat; commonly called a cold

8. ____ Chronic inflammatory disease that occurs when the respiratory system reacts strongly to irritants, infection, cold air, or to allergens; causes coughing and difficulty breathing

9. ____ Development of abnormal cells or tumors in the lungs

10. ____ Condition in which the bronchial tubes are abnormally enlarged; causes chronic coughing

(A) Asthma

(B) Bronchiectasis

(C) Lung cancer

(D) Tuberculosis (TB)

(E) Upper respiratory infection (URI)

6. Describe common diseases and disorders of the endocrine system

Multiple Choice

1. Diabetes is a condition in which the pancreas does not produce enough or properly use
   (A) Insulin
   (B) Glucose
   (C) Growth hormones
   (D) Adrenaline

2. Sugars collecting in the blood cause problems with
   (A) Breathing
   (B) Circulation
   (C) Pulse rate
   (D) Blood pressure

3. Type 1 diabetes
   (A) Continues throughout a person's life
   (B) Is most common in the elderly
   (C) Is treated with surgery
   (D) Does not require a change of diet

4. Changes in the circulatory system from diabetes can cause
   (A) Hair loss
   (B) Heart attack and stroke
   (C) Opportunistic infections
   (D) COPD

5. The most common form of diabetes is
   (A) Pre-diabetes
   (B) Gestational diabetes
   (C) Type 1 diabetes
   (D) Type 2 diabetes

6. Poor circulation and impaired wound healing may result in
   (A) Urinary tract infections
   (B) Cancer
   (C) Gangrene
   (D) AIDS

7. Gangrene can lead to
   (A) Loss of bowel control
   (B) Paralysis
   (C) Congestive heart failure
   (D) Amputation

8. What condition occurs when a person's blood glucose level is above normal but not high enough for a diagnosis of Type 2 diabetes?
   (A) Gestational diabetes
   (B) Type 1 diabetes
   (C) Pre-diabetes
   (D) Hyperglycemia

9. Careful _____ care is vitally important for people with diabetes.
   (A) Foot
   (B) Hair
   (C) Facial
   (D) Mouth

Short Answer

10. How much should a diabetic resident eat of what is served?

    _____

    _____

    _____

    _____

11. Why is careful foot care so important for a diabetic resident?

    _____

    _____

    _____

    _____

    _____

    _____

12. What is hyperthyroidism?

    _____

    _____

    _____

    _____

13. What is hypothyroidism?

    _____

    _____

    _____

    _____

7. Describe common diseases and disorders of the reproductive system

True or False

1. _____ Gonorrhea can be treated with antibiotics and is easier to detect in men than in women.

2. _____ People with herpes always experience repeated outbreaks.

3. _____ Condoms can reduce the chances of being infected or passing on some STDs and STIs.

4. _____ Gonorrhea can cause sterility in both men and women.

5. _____ Symptoms of chlamydia include yellow or white discharge from the penis or vagina and a burning sensation during urination.

6. _____ Chlamydia cannot be treated with antibiotics.

7. _____ If left untreated, syphilis can cause brain damage or death.

8. _____ Most women infected with gonorrhea show many early symptoms.

9. _____ Benign prostatic hypertrophy is a fairly common disorder that occurs in both women and men as they age.

10. _____ STDs and STIs can only be transmitted by sexual intercourse.

11. _____ Herpes is caused by a virus and cannot be treated with antibiotics.

12. _____ Chancres, or open sores, that develop on the penis make it easier for syphilis to be detected in men than in women.

13. _____ Penicillin can be used to treat syphilis.

14. _____ Vaginitis can be caused by bacteria, protozoa, or fungus.

15. _____ Before having a vaginal douche, the woman will be placed in the prone position.

8. Describe common diseases and disorders of the immune and lymphatic systems

True or False

1. _____ HIV and AIDS are the same thing.

2. _____ HIV can only be transmitted sexually.

3. _____ The first stage of HIV infection involves symptoms similar to flu.

4. _____ There is no known cure for AIDS.

5. _____ AIDS dementia complex occurs in the early stages of AIDS.

Short Answer

6. List five signs and symptoms of HIV infection and AIDS.

_____

_____

_____

_____

_____

_____

_____

_____

_____

7. What is an opportunistic infection?

_____

_____

_____

_____

_____

Multiple Choice

8. Care for the person who has HIV or AIDS should focus on
   (A) Helping to find a cure for HIV
   (B) Preventing visits from friends and family
   (C) Providing relief of symptoms and preventing infection
   (D) Making judgments about the resident

9. If your resident with AIDS has a poor appetite, you should
   (A) Give them an over-the-counter appetite stimulant
   (B) Serve familiar and favorite foods
   (C) Let them know that if the resident does not eat, he might die
   (D) Discuss this with the resident's friends and family and see what they recommend doing

10. AIDS residents who have infections of the mouth and esophagus may need to eat food that is
    (A) Spicy
    (B) Low in acid
    (C) Dry
    (D) Steaming hot

11. Someone who has nausea and vomiting should
    (A) Eat mostly dairy products
    (B) Eat high-fat and spicy foods
    (C) Drink liquids and eat salty foods
    (D) Reduce liquid intake

12. The "BRAT" diet is helpful for
    (A) Diarrhea
    (B) Weight gain
    (C) Nausea and vomiting
    (D) Headaches

13. Fluids are important for residents who have diarrhea because
    (A) Diarrhea rapidly depletes the body of fluids.
    (B) Diarrhea can be prevented by drinking a lot of fluids.
    (C) Fluid intake is not important for a person who has diarrhea.
    (D) Diarrhea causes HIV infection.

14. The following is helpful in dealing with neuropathy
    (A) Wrapping feet tightly in bandages
    (B) Wearing tight shoes
    (C) Using a bed cradle
    (D) Tucking in bed sheets tightly

15. Legal rights regarding HIV include
    (A) A person with HIV can be fired if the employer did not know that information before the person was hired.
    (B) Employers can force new employees to be tested for HIV/AIDS upon hiring them.
    (C) A nursing assistant can share a resident's diagnosis of HIV/AIDS with anyone the resident may come into contact with.
    (D) HIV test results are confidential and cannot be shared with anyone.

Fill in the Blank
Fill in the blanks with the words listed below.

Benign   Malignant
Cancer   Tumor
Cure

16. _____ is a general term used to describe many types of malignant tumors.

17. A _____ is a cluster of abnormally growing cells.

18. _____ tumors grow slowly in local areas and are considered noncancerous.

19. _____ tumors grow rapidly and invade surrounding tissues.

20. There is no known _____ for cancer.

Short Answer
Mark an "X" beside the American Cancer Society's warning signs of cancer.

21. _____ Change in bowel or bladder habits
22. _____ Difficulty breathing
23. _____ Dizziness
24. _____ Thickening or lump in breast
25. _____ Memory loss
26. _____ Recent change in wart or mole
27. _____ Pain
28. _____ Nagging cough or hoarseness
29. _____ Indigestion or difficulty swallowing
30. _____ Nausea or vomiting
31. _____ Sweet, fruity breath odor
32. _____ Sore that does not heal
33. _____ Unusual bleeding or discharge
34. _____ Headache

Name: _____

35. The first line of defense for malignant tumors of the skin, breast, bladder, colon, rectum, stomach, and muscle is
    (A) Surgery
    (B) Homeopathic pills
    (C) Radiation
    (D) Herbal remedies

36. Nausea, vomiting, diarrhea, hair loss, and decreased resistance to infection are all side effects of which treatment?
    (A) Surgery
    (B) Chemotherapy
    (C) Diet and exercise
    (D) Herbal remedies

37. This treatment method uses medications to destroy cancer cells and limit the rate of cell growth
    (A) Homeopathic pills
    (B) Chemotherapy
    (C) Radiation
    (D) Herbal remedies

38. This treatment method involves removing as much of the tumor as possible to prevent cancer from spreading
    (A) Surgery
    (B) Chemotherapy
    (C) Radiation
    (D) Herbal remedies

39. This treatment method kills normal and abnormal cells in a limited area, sometimes causing skin to become sore, irritated, or burned
    (A) Surgery
    (B) Chemotherapy
    (C) Radiation
    (D) Herbal remedies

40. To help promote good nutrition, you can do the following
    (A) Use metal utensils for residents
    (B) Serve a variety of foods that are high in nutrition
    (C) Restrict nutritional supplements
    (D) Serve foods with little nutritional content

41. If your resident is experiencing pain, you should
    (A) Assist with comfort measures
    (B) Not report it
    (C) Give the resident pain medication
    (D) Tell the resident that you cannot do anything about it

42. Which of the following is a good idea for communicating with a resident who has cancer?
    (A) Insist that the resident tell you what he or she is going through.
    (B) Tell the resident about any new medications that he or she should take.
    (C) If the resident is worried, tell him or her "It'll all be fine."
    (D) Listen to the resident if he or she feels like talking.

9. Identify community resources for residents who are ill

Short Answer

List three types of organizations that provide services and support for people who are ill and their families.

_____

_____

_____

_____

_____

_____

19

Confusion, Dementia, and Alzheimer's Disease

1. Describe normal changes of aging in the brain

Multiple Choice

1. The ability to think logically and quickly is called
   (A) Cognition
   (B) Dementia
   (C) Awareness
   (D) Respiration

2. Cognitive impairment affects
   (A) Social security reform
   (B) Motor skills
   (C) Concentration and memory
   (D) Diet

3. Nursing assistants can help elderly residents with memory loss by
   (A) Doing as much as possible for them
   (B) Encouraging them to make lists of things to remember
   (C) Reminding them every time they forget something
   (D) Telling them to think as hard as they can

2. Discuss confusion and delirium

Short Answer

1. What 10 actions can you take when you are helping care for a resident who is confused?

   _____

   _____

   _____

   _____

   _____

   _____

   _____

   _____

   _____

   _____

   _____

   _____

   _____

2. Name four possible causes of delirium.

   _____

   _____

   _____

   _____

3. Describe dementia and define related terms

True or False

1. _____ Dementia is the loss of mental abilities such as thinking, remembering, reasoning, and communicating.

2. _____ Dementia is a normal part of aging.

3. _____ An irreversible disease can be cured with medication and surgery.

4. _____ Degenerative diseases get continually worse, causing a greater loss of health and abilities.

5. _____ Alzheimer's disease is a common cause of dementia.

4. Describe Alzheimer's disease and identify its stages

True or False

1. _____ Alzheimer's disease is the most common cause of dementia in the elderly.

2. _____ Men are more likely to have Alzheimer's disease than women are.

3. _____ Alzheimer's disease is a normal part of aging, and everyone eventually will have it.

4. _____ Alzheimer's disease causes tangled nerve fibers and protein deposits to form in the brain, eventually causing dementia.

5. _____ There is no cure for Alzheimer's disease.

6. _____ Diagnosing Alzheimer's disease is usually a simple and quick procedure.

7. _____ Symptoms of Alzheimer's disease typically appear suddenly.

8. _____ Each person with Alzheimer's disease will show different signs at different times.

9. _____ Skills that a person has learned recently are usually kept longer after onset of Alzheimer's disease.

10. _____ Alzheimer's disease victims will eventually need constant care.

11. _____ Encouraging residents with Alzheimer's disease to keep their minds and bodies active may help slow the disease.

5. Identify personal attitudes helpful in caring for residents with Alzheimer's disease

Scenarios
Read each scenario below. State which of the personal attitudes from the learning objective would be helpful in each situation and explain why.

1. You have been working all day and are very tired. You have a headache and have not had time to eat a decent meal. You do not know how you will summon the energy to come back to work tomorrow and take care of Mrs. Jones, a resident with Alzheimer's whose behavior has been very challenging lately.

_____

_____

_____

_____

_____

_____

_____

_____

2. Ms. Yancy has Alzheimer's. She is still in the very early stages of the disease, but she gets very depressed when she thinks about what will happen to her later. She has not opened up to you about things that she likes to do or talk about, and you would like her to be more comfortable with you. You notice that when her daughter comes to visit her, she always brightens up a bit.

_____

_____

_____

_____

_____

_____

3. A resident becomes very depressed one morning while you are helping him shave. He tells you that you are lucky that you do not need someone to help you do everyday tasks. He says that he hopes you appreciate your good health.

_____

_____

_____

_____

_____

_____

4. A resident tells you that you are stupid and that she hates having to see you every morning. She says that she does not know how anyone was foolish enough to hire you and that she will be complaining to the nurse about you every day until you are fired.

_____

_____

_____

_____

_____

_____

5. On Monday afternoon, Mr. Kotter was lively and friendly. He said that he was looking forward to a Tuesday afternoon card game he was going to have with his two best friends. On Tuesday when you stop by his room to get him ready to go to the card game, he says he hates cards and he does not like any of the people who are playing. He would prefer to go for a walk by himself.

_____

_____

_____

_____

_____

_____

_____

6. List strategies for better communication with residents with Alzheimer's disease

Scenarios
Read each scenario below and state an appropriate response for each.

1. Mrs. Hays, a resident with AD, has awakened from her nap and does not recognize her room or anyone around her.

_____

_____

_____

_____

_____

2. Blake, an NA, has been trying to give Mr. Collins, a resident with AD, a bath. Mr. Collins has become agitated and is asking Blake, "Who are you?" over and over again, although Blake has already identified himself twice.

_____

_____

_____

_____

_____

3. Mrs. Hays has been telling Blake a story about her niece. She is showing him a necklace that her niece had given her as a gift. She is having trouble remembering the word "necklace," and is getting upset.

_____

_____

_____

_____

_____

_____

_____

_____

4. Blake is helping Mr. Collins get ready to go to dinner. Blake asks him to put his shoes on, but Mr. Collins does not understand what Blake wants him to do.

_____

_____

_____

_____

_____

_____

_____

_____

Multiple Choice

5. When communicating with a resident with AD, you should
   (A) Approach the resident from behind.
   (B) Stand as close as you are comfortable to the resident.
   (C) Communicate in a loud, busy place.
   (D) Speak slowly, using a lower tone of voice than normal.

6. If a resident is frightened or anxious, which of the following should you do?
   (A) Check your body language so you do not appear tense or hurried.
   (B) Turn up the television or radio to try to distract the resident.
   (C) Use complex sentences.
   (D) Give multiple instructions at one time so that the resident has time to absorb them.

7. If a resident perseverates, this means he or she is
   (A) Repeating words, phrases, questions, or actions
   (B) Suggesting words that sound correct
   (C) Hallucinating
   (D) Gesturing instead of speaking to you

8. If the resident does not remember how to perform basic tasks, you should
   (A) Do everything for him or her
   (B) Encourage the resident to do what he or she can
   (C) Skip explaining each activity
   (D) Say "don't" as often as you feel is necessary

7. Explain general principles that will help assist residents with personal care

Word Search
Fill in the blanks below and find your answers in the word search.

1. Make a _____ and stick to it.

2. Being _____ is important for residents who are confused and easily upset.

3. Promote _____. This will help residents _____.

4. Take good care of _____, both _____ and physically.

```
x m o i u m z r k o s r c c
p t j z m u e s t u e o t g
o i f d l m r n m q p j u z
y o u r s e l f t e t n c r
b y r n m p f e n a u d r o
j n w z a w r z e g l k k u
r p m d s a e b t v o l e t
u q n d c n y l s e c h y i
i w d f x k e f i e i m f n
l u l i a f h x s j h b b e
z e n i m a o z n h q a e n
s x p j f a w t o p q c n o
k c t g b v n g c m v a l z
c d v d c d z m e w a t c v
```

8. List and describe interventions for problems with common activities of daily living (ADLs)

Short Answer
For each of the following statements, write "good idea" if the statement is a good idea for residents with Alzheimer's disease, and "bad idea" if the statement is a bad idea.

1. Use nonslip mats, tub seats, and hand holds to ensure safety during bathing.

   _____

2. Always bathe the resident at the same time every day, even if he or she is agitated.

   _____

3. Break tasks down into simple steps, explaining one step at a time.

   _____

4. Do not attempt to groom the resident, since he or she may not enjoy this.

   _____

5. Choose clothes that are simple to put on.

   _____

6. If the resident is incontinent, do not give him or her fluids.

   _____

7. Mark the restroom with a sign or picture as a reminder of when to use it and where it is.

   _____

8. Check the skin regularly for signs of irritation.

   _____

9. Follow Standard Precautions when caring for the resident.

   _____

10. Do not encourage exercise, as this will make the resident more agitated.

    _____

11. Serve finger foods if the resident tends to wander during meals.

    _____

12. Schedule meals at the same time every day.

    _____

13. Serve new kinds of foods as often as possible to stimulate the resident.

    _____

14. Put only one kind of food on the plate at a time.

    _____

15. Put food on white dishes without a pattern.

    _____

16. Do not encourage independence, as this can lead to aggressive behavior.

    _____

17. Protect privacy by keeping resident covered, even if he is unaware.

    _____

18. Reward positive behavior with smiles, hugs, warm touches, and thanks.

    _____

9. List and describe interventions for common difficult behaviors related to Alzheimer's disease

Scenarios

For each description below, identify the behavior and state one way of dealing with it.

1. Mrs. Donne gets upset at about nine o'clock every night. She repeatedly asks for snacks or drinks and refuses to go to bed.

    _____

    _____

    _____

    _____

    _____

2. Mr. Grayson is playing chess with a friend and becomes angry when he loses. He shoves his friend, and when the nurse approaches them, he tells her he is going to hit her.

    _____

    _____

    _____

    _____

    _____

3. Mr. Cayne gets very upset every time he sees the president on television. He yells at the screen and tells everyone how poor a state our country has gotten into.

    _____

    _____

    _____

    _____

    _____

4. Ms. Hobbes used to enjoy talking to people and reading, but lately she does not seem to enjoy anything. She sleeps most of the day and never talks to anyone unless she is asked to.

    _____

    _____

    _____

    _____

    _____

    _____

5. Whenever Mr. Henderson does not like what is being served for dinner, he bangs on the table with his fists and shouts about how much he hates his food. When people try to get him to stop, he only seems to grow louder.

    _____

    _____

    _____

    _____

    _____

6. Mr. Ryan is walking around the facility asking everyone he meets what time it is. Even though he has been told several times, he still seems unsatisfied and keeps asking the question.

    _____

    _____

    _____

    _____

    _____

    _____

7. About an hour before dinner every night, Ms. Lordes starts walking up and down the hall as quickly as she can. She does not speak to or acknowledge anyone else while she is doing this.

_____
_____
_____
_____
_____

8. Whenever a female resident comes into the television room, Mr. Ratcliffe tells her that he loves her and starts removing his clothes. If she stays in the room long enough, he will ask her to take off her clothes, too.

_____
_____
_____
_____
_____

9. Mrs. Leone loves the color red. She has a lot of red clothing that she enjoys wearing. Whenever she sees a piece of red clothing, even in another resident's room, she picks it up and takes it back to her room.

_____
_____
_____
_____
_____

10. Mr. Gordon tells you that his wife has just called him on the phone. She is coming to pick him up and they are going to dinner at the place they went on their first date. You know that his wife has been dead for several years, and their favorite restaurant has long since closed down.

_____
_____
_____
_____
_____
_____
_____

10. Describe creative therapies for residents with Alzheimer's disease

Scenarios
For each situation described below, identify the therapy that the nursing assistant is using.

1. Ms. Lee misses her husband, who has been dead for ten years, very much. Lisa, an NA who works with her, always asks about her life with her husband and what it was like. Ms. Lee seems to enjoy telling Lisa stories about what they did when they were young and how happy she was when they were together.

_____
_____
_____
_____
_____
_____

2. Mr. Elking tells Lisa that he has a date with Nora, the pretty girl who lives across the street. He is going to take her dancing and out to a movie. Lisa knows that Nora lived in his neighborhood when he was a teenager and he has not seen her for years, and that Mr. Elking rarely gets out of bed. Instead of correcting him, Lisa asks him what kind of movie they are going to see and what he thinks he should wear.

_____

_____

_____

_____

_____

3. Mr. Aiken sometimes gets depressed, especially in the evenings. Lisa knows that he loves classical music, so she starts playing it for him in the evenings a little before he usually starts feeling sad. He sorts through albums and places them in stacks.

_____

_____

_____

_____

_____

4. Mrs. Connor is in the first stage of AD. Lately she has been having trouble remembering which month of the year it is. Lisa brings her a colorful calendar that has a different scene for each month to help her remember.

_____

_____

_____

_____

_____

11. Discuss how Alzheimer's disease may affect the family

Short Answer

1. Why might it be difficult for families of people who have AD?

_____

_____

_____

_____

_____

2. What two major resources affect the ability of residents' families to cope with AD?

_____

_____

_____

_____

12. Identify community resources available to people with Alzheimer's disease and their families

Short Answer

List four resources people with AD and their families can turn to in times of need.

_____

_____

_____

_____

_____

20

Mental Health and Mental Illness

1. Identify seven characteristics of mental health

Short Answer

1. Define mental health.

_____

_____

_____

_____

_____

2. List five characteristics of a person who is mentally healthy.

_____

_____

_____

_____

_____

_____

_____

_____

_____

_____

2. Identify four causes of mental illness

True or False

1. _____ Signs and symptoms of mental illness include confusion, disorientation, agitation, and anxiety.

2. _____ A situation response may be triggered by severe changes in the environment.

3. _____ A mentally healthy person cannot experience a situation response.

4. _____ Mental illness can be brought on by substance abuse or a chemical imbalance.

5. _____ The building blocks of mental health are self-respect and self-worth.

6. _____ Traumatic experiences early in life do not cause mental illness.

7. _____ Mental illness cannot be inherited.

8. _____ Extreme stress may result in mental illness.

9. _____ Mental illness is a disease.

3. Distinguish between fact and fallacy concerning mental illness

True or False

1. _____ A fallacy is a false belief.

2. _____ People who are mentally ill have the power to control their illness if they want to.

3. _____ People who are mentally ill do not want to get well.

4. _____ Mental illness is a disease just like any physical illness.

5. _____ People who are mentally ill often cannot control their emotions or responses to people and situations.

6. _____ Mental retardation is a type of mental illness.

4. Explain the connection between mental and physical wellness

Short Answer

Briefly describe why mental health is important to physical health.

_____

_____

_____

_____

_____

_____

_____

_____

_____

_____

5. List guidelines for communicating with mentally ill residents

Labeling
Fill in the blanks to show how to practice good communication skills with mentally ill residents.

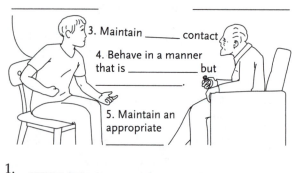

1. Stand or sit with a posture that says you're _____

2. Practice _____

3. Maintain _____ contact

4. Behave in a manner that is _____ but _____.

5. Maintain an appropriate

1. _____

2. _____

3. _____

4. _____

5. _____

6. Identify and define common defense mechanisms

Short Answer
Read each description below and identify the defense mechanism that is being used.

1. When Aaron's mother yells at him for breaking a vase in the living room, he goes into his room and yells at his stuffed bear.

   _____

   _____

2. When Gia was 10, she was very badly injured in a car accident. She was in the hospital for almost three months, but now she cannot remember anything at all about that time.

   _____

   _____

3. When Mark accuses his little sister Sarah of having a crush on the boy who sits next to her in class, she blushes and cries, "I do not!"

   _____

   _____

4. When Esther was 42, her husband died of lung cancer. After his death, she got out the quilt she used to sleep in as a child and curled up in bed with it for days.

   _____

   _____

5. Wayne is fixing a leaky sink in the bathroom. When his wife teases him about taking a long time to fix it, he replies, "It's not my fault. I can't concentrate on anything with you bothering me all the time."

   _____

6. Martin's girlfriend promised to go out with him on Thursday night, but she forgets and goes out with her sister instead. Martin is annoyed, but does not say anything to her. When he goes out with his friends that night, he tells them that she is mad at him.

_____

_____

_____

7. Describe the symptoms of anxiety, depression, and schizophrenia

Fill in the Blank
Using the words below, complete each of the following statements. Each word is used only once.

Anxiety   Hallucinations

Apathy   Major

Bipolar   Obsessive compulsive

Claustrophobia   Phobia

Delusions   Schizophrenia

1. Lack of interest in activities is called
_____.

2. An intense form of anxiety, such as fear of flying, is called a
_____.

3. Illusions that a person sees or hears are called _____.

4. When a person washes his hands over and over again as a way of dealing with anxiety, this type of behavior is called

_____ disorder.

5. _____ is uneasiness or fear, often about a situation or condition.

6. _____ depression may cause a person to lose interest in everything he once cared about.

7. Fear of being in a confined space, such as an elevator, is called
_____.

8. _____ is a brain disorder that affects a person's ability to think and communicate clearly.

9. _____ disorder causes a person to swing from profound depression to extreme activity.

10. _____ are persistent false beliefs, such as thinking that other people can read one's thoughts.

8. Explain how mental illness is treated

True or False

1. _____ Mental illness cannot be treated.

2. _____ Medication and psychotherapy are commonly used to treat mental illness.

3. _____ Nursing assistants are responsible for giving mentally ill residents their medication.

4. _____ Medication can allow the mentally ill to function more completely.

5. _____ Electroconvulsive (shock) treatment (EST) is not commonly used to treat mental illness.

9. Explain your role in caring for residents who are mentally ill

Short Answer

List three special responsibilities that you will have when caring for mentally ill residents.

_____

_____

_____

_____

_____

_____

_____

_____

Name: _____

10. Identify important observations that should be made and reported

True or False

1. _____ It is important to report to the nurse if a mentally ill resident stops taking his or her medication.

2. _____ You do not need to worry about a mentally ill resident discussing suicide if he or she is just joking about it.

3. _____ You should report to the nurse if a mentally ill resident has an extremely happy reaction to bad news.

11. List the signs of substance abuse

Crossword
Fill in the blanks below and use your answers to complete the crossword puzzle.

Across

2. Loss of _____

4. Odor of _____, liquor, or other substances on breath or clothes

7. Frequent

_____

9. Unexplained changes in

_____

signs

Down

1. Red eyes, _____ loss

3. Changes in

_____,

moodiness, strange behavior

5. Need for _____

6. _____

or memory loss

8. Reduced sense of

_____

Multiple Choice

10. Circle all of the following substances that can be abused
    (A) Alcohol
    (B) Cigarettes
    (C) Decongestants
    (D) Diet aids
    (E) Illegal drugs
    (F) Glue
    (G) Paint
    (H) Prescription medicine

11. Your resident has been acting a little strangely lately. She gets upset very easily and her eyes are always red. She does not eat much, and sometimes you can smell alcohol on her breath, even in the morning. What should you do?

(A) Confront your resident about what you have noticed.

(B) Call Alcoholics Anonymous.

(C) Document your observations and report them to the nurse.

(D) Search the resident's dresser and side table for alcohol and throw away whatever you find.

Name: _____

21

Rehabilitation and Restorative Care

1. Discuss rehabilitation and restorative care

Multiple Choice

1. What is the goal of rehabilitation?
   (A) To restore the person's intelligence
   (B) To restore the person to the highest possible level of functioning
   (C) To reach the level of functionality of a normal person
   (D) To cure a disease

2. Which care team member establishes the goals of care for rehabilitation?
   (A) Doctor
   (B) Social worker
   (C) Nursing assistant
   (D) Counselor

3. What is the goal of restorative services?
   (A) To diagnose disease
   (B) To create new infection prevention policies
   (C) To keep the resident at the level achieved by rehabilitation
   (D) To get the family to visit more often

Short Answer

4. Rehabilitation will be used for many of your residents, but particularly for those who have suffered what three incidents?

_____

_____

_____

_____

_____

5. Why are nursing assistants a very important part of the restorative care team?

_____

_____

_____

_____

_____

_____

_____

True or False

6. _____ Ignore any setbacks a resident experiences so he or she does not become discouraged.

7. _____ Your reactions and attitudes really do not affect a resident's progress.

8. _____ If you can do a task faster than your resident, you should do it yourself.

9. _____ Do not report any decline in a resident's ability.

10. _____ Family members and residents will take cues from you on how to behave.

11. _____ Tasks are less overwhelming when they are broken down into small steps.

12. _____ It is important to report any signs of depression or mood changes in a resident.

13. _____ All residents will enjoy being encouraged in an obvious way.

14. _____ When residents are demanding or irritating, it is OK to unplug their call light until their attitude improves.

2. Describe the importance of promoting independence and list ways exercise improves health

Short Answer

1. List nine problems that can result from inactivity and immobility.

_____

_____

_____

_____

_____

_____

_____

_____

2. What does regular ambulation and exercise help improve?

_____

_____

_____

_____

_____

3. Describe assistive devices and equipment

Multiple Choice

1. Assistive devices help residents
    (A) Fight infection
    (B) Make decisions about care
    (C) Perform their activities of daily living (ADLs)
    (D) Communicate

2. Supportive devices are used to assist residents with
    (A) Personal care
    (B) Ambulation
    (C) Burns
    (D) Vital signs

3. Safety devices are used for
    (A) Preventing accidents
    (B) Sleeping
    (C) Ambulation
    (D) Incontinence

Short Answer

4. Choose an adaptive device from Figure 21-2 in the textbook that you did not choose for the Chapter Review. Describe how it might help a resident who is recovering from or adapting to a physical condition.

_____

_____

_____

_____

_____

_____

4. Explain guidelines for maintaining proper body alignment

Fill in the Blank

1. Observe principles of _____. Remember that proper alignment is based on a straight _____. _____ or rolled or folded _____ may be needed to support the small of the back and raise the knees or head in the supine position.

2. Keep body parts in natural _____. In a natural hand position, the fingers are slightly _____. Use _____ to keep covers from resting on feet in the supine position.

3. Prevent external rotation of _____. Change _____ frequently to prevent muscle stiffness and pressure sores. Every _____ hours is usually adequate.

5. Explain care guidelines for prosthetic devices

True or False

1. _____ Wearing gloves is unnecessary when caring for an artificial eye.

2. _____ Prostheses are expensive, specially-fitted pieces of equipment.

3. _____ Artificial eyes are held in by a special type of glue.

4. _____ A prosthesis is a device that replaces a body part that is missing or deformed because of an accident, injury, illness, or birth defect.

5. _____ Artificial eyes should be rinsed in rubbing alcohol.

6. _____ If a prosthesis is broken or does not fit properly, it is best to try to repair it before reporting it to the nurse.

7. _____ When observing the skin on the stump, it is important to check for signs of skin breakdown caused by pressure and abrasion.

6. Describe how to assist with range of motion exercises

Matching

For each of the following terms, write the letter of the correct definition from the list below.

1. _____ active assisted range of motion

2. _____ active range of motion

3. _____ passive range of motion

4. _____ range of motion

(A) Exercises performed by the resident with some assistance and support

(B) Exercises used by residents who are not able to move on their own

(C) Exercises that put a particular joint through its full arc of motion

(D) Exercises performed by the resident himself, using his own muscle power

Labeling

For each of the following illustrations, put the correct term of the body movement.

5. _____
_____
_____

6. _____
_____
_____

7. _____
_____
_____

8. _____
_____
_____

9. _____
_____
_____

10. _____
_____
_____

11. _____
_____
_____

12. _____
_____
_____

Name: _____

Multiple Choice

13. In what order should ROM exercises be done?
    (A) Start from the feet and work up
    (B) Start from the head and work down
    (C) The arms and legs should be exercised first
    (D) The arms and legs should be exercised last

14. If a resident reports pain during ROM exercises, you should
    (A) Continue with the exercises as planned
    (B) Continue, but perform the motion that caused pain more gently
    (C) Stop the exercises and report the pain to the nurse
    (D) Stop the motion for one minute before starting again

15. How many times will you repeat each exercise while assisting with range of motion?
    (A) At least 6 times
    (B) At least 10 times
    (C) At least 12 times
    (D) At least 3 times

7. Describe the benefits of deep breathing exercises

Short Answer

What can deep breathing exercises help?

_____

_____

_____

_____

_____

_____

_____

_____

22

Special Care Skills

1. Understand the types of residents who are in a subacute setting

True or False

1. _____ A subacute setting is a special unit for those who need more care than most long-term facilities can give.

2. _____ Hospitals can provide subacute care, but skilled nursing facilities cannot.

3. _____ People who have had surgery, have chronic illnesses, or require dialysis or complex wound care may need subacute care.

4. _____ A mechanical ventilator is a machine that assists with or replaces breathing when a person cannot breathe on his own.

2. Discuss reasons for and types of surgery

Multiple Choice

1. Which type of surgery must be performed for health reasons, but is not an emergency?
   (A) Elective
   (B) Urgent
   (C) Emergency
   (D) Plastic

2. _____ surgery is unexpected and unscheduled and must be performed immediately to save a life or limb.
   (A) Elective
   (B) Urgent
   (C) Emergency
   (D) Plastic

3. Which type of surgery is chosen by the patient and is planned in advance?
   (A) Elective
   (B) Urgent
   (C) Emergency
   (D) Non-elective

4. Which type of anesthesia is injected directly into the surgical site or area and is used for minor surgical procedures?
   (A) Local anesthesia
   (B) General anesthesia
   (C) Full body anesthesia
   (D) Intravenous anesthesia

5. An epidural is an example of this type of anesthesia.
   (A) Regional anesthesia
   (B) General anesthesia
   (C) Local anesthesia
   (D) Intravenous anesthesia

3. Discuss preoperative care

True or False

1. _____ Before a person has surgery, the doctor will most likely not tell him or her what to expect because that may frighten the person too much.

2. _____ People who are going to have surgery often experience anxiety, fear, worry, and sadness.

3. _____ A nursing assistant can help a person who is worried about surgery by avoiding the person until the surgery is over.

4. _____ If a person has an order for "NPO" before surgery, this means that he or she cannot not have food or drink, except for water.

134

Name: _____

5. ____ A nursing assistant's duties may include making sure that the person's identification bracelet is accurate and on the wrist or ankle prior to transport.

4. Describe postoperative care

Short Answer

1. What are three goals of postoperative care?

_____

_____

_____

2. What are the concerns and possible complications to watch for after a person has surgery?

_____

_____

_____

_____

3. What type of equipment might you be asked to gather while a resident is in recovery after surgery?

_____

_____

_____

_____

4. List ten tasks that you may be required to do for postoperative care.

_____

_____

_____

_____

_____

_____

_____

_____

_____

_____

_____

_____

_____

5. List ten signs and symptoms of postoperative complications that you need to observe for and report.

_____

_____

_____

_____

_____

_____

_____

5. List care guidelines for pulse oximetry

Multiple Choice

1. Pulse oximetry is commonly used for people who are
   (A) Diabetic
   (B) Incontinent
   (C) Returning from surgery
   (D) Demented

2. A pulse oximeter measures
   (A) Blood oxygen level
   (B) Swelling of the extremities
   (C) Weight
   (D) Medication level

3. The pulse oximeter's sensor is usually clipped on a person's
   (A) Knee
   (B) Elbow
   (C) Chin
   (D) Finger

4. The sensor uses_____ to measure blood oxygen level.
   (A) Light
   (B) Sound
   (C) Chemicals
   (D) Vibrations

5. A normal blood oxygen level is usually between
   (A) 25% - 40%
   (B) 40% - 60%
   (C) 60% - 70%
   (D) 95% - 100%

6. Which of the following should be reported to the nurse regarding pulse oximetry?
   (A) The oximeter displays the blood oxygen level.
   (B) The resident is resting comfortably.
   (C) The alarm sounds.
   (D) The resident requests extra pillows.

6. Describe telemetry and list care guidelines

Word Search
Fill in the blanks below and find your answers in the word search.

1. Telemetry is used to measure the heart _____ and

   _____

   on a continuous basis.

2. Wires are attached to the

   _____

   with sticky pads or patches.

3. Report to the nurse if the pads become

   _____

   or soiled.

4. If the _____
   sounds, notify the nurse.

5. Check _____
   signs as ordered.

6. Check the skin around the pads for sores, redness, or _____.

```
e  t  h  h  z  v  s  f  b  r  i  b  q  u
u  s  s  m  a  g  r  z  n  z  g  l  z  p
s  g  m  b  x  j  x  o  j  f  r  q  j  y
v  l  e  h  b  d  y  s  k  g  a  y  x  t
g  w  v  i  t  a  l  l  u  a  z  a  c  i
r  i  e  d  w  y  m  p  i  d  w  t  k  m
g  l  i  t  e  r  h  f  o  u  g  q  o  g
n  o  i  t  a  t  i  r  r  i  w  e  g  r
i  w  g  l  s  r  w  o  a  j  w  s  i  l
s  z  a  e  c  k  j  y  x  j  v  s  h  i
t  t  h  b  v  b  q  k  b  v  h  q  y  r
k  c  w  y  z  x  e  n  u  b  a  i  s  m
o  m  a  n  u  z  f  z  j  o  t  z  d  q
v  z  m  q  v  j  l  l  n  a  n  h  y  d
```

7. Explain artificial airways and list care guidelines

Short Answer

1. List three situations in which an artificial airway might be necessary.

   _____

   _____

   _____

   _____

   _____

2. What is a tracheostomy?

   _____

   _____

   _____

   _____

3. List four guidelines for working with residents with artificial airways.

   _____

   _____

   _____

   _____

   _____

   _____

   _____

8. Discuss care for a resident with a tracheostomy

True or False

1. _____ A tracheostomy is always permanent.

2. _____ It may be difficult for the resident to talk after first having a tracheostomy placed.

3. _____ Cancer, infection, and severe neck or mouth injuries are some reasons why a tracheostomy may be necessary.

4. _____ Gurgling sounds are normal due to the placement in the neck and do not need to be reported to the nurse.

5. _____ Nursing assistants do not perform tracheostomy care or suctioning.

6. _____ Shortness of breath or trouble breathing should be reported right away.

7. _____ Residents with tracheostomies are prone to respiratory infections.

8. _____ To help prevent infection when working with residents with tracheostomies, wash your hands often.

9. List care guidelines for residents requiring mechanical ventilation

Crossword Puzzle

Across

2. Residents will not be able to

_____

while on the mechanical ventilator because air will no longer reach the larynx.

4. Give regular, careful skin care to prevent _____ sores.

8. An agent or drug that helps calm and soothe a person and may cause sleep is called a

_____.

9. Answer the _____ promptly.

Down

1. _____

your hands often when working with residents on mechanical ventilators.

2. Being on a ventilator has been compared to breathing through a _____.

5. Mechanical ventilation is using a machine to assist with or replace

_____ when a person is unable to do this on his own.

7. Enter the room _____ so that the resident can see you; this can lessen anxiety and reassure the person.

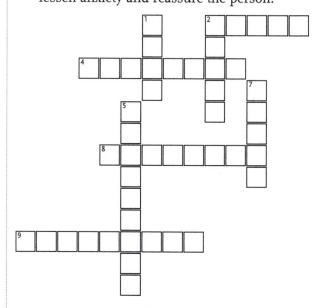

10. Describe suctioning and list signs of respiratory distress

True or False

1. _____ Suctioning is needed when a person cannot remove mucus and secretions from the lungs on his own.

2. _____ Suctioning is normally a non-sterile procedure.

3. _____ The nursing assistant is responsible for suctioning.

4. _____ A portable pump may be used to suction the resident.

5. _____ One sign of respiratory distress is a gurgling sound of secretions.

6. _____ If a person is flaring his nostrils, he may be in respiratory distress.

7. _____ Vital signs, especially respiratory rate, should be monitored closely.

11. Describe chest tubes and explain related care

Multiple Choice

1. Chest tubes are inserted during a _____ procedure.
   (A) Sterile
   (B) Non-sterile
   (C) Personal care
   (D) Catheterization

2. Chest tubes drain air, blood, or fluid from
   (A) The heart
   (B) The brain
   (C) The pleural cavity
   (D) The esophagus

3. Chest tubes may be required for
   (A) Vaginitis
   (B) Eczema
   (C) Nutritional deficiencies
   (D) Surgery or injuries

4. The system must be
   (A) Recycled
   (B) Permanent
   (C) Airtight
   (D) Frozen

5. The drainage system must be kept _____ the level of the resident's chest.
   (A) Above
   (B) Below
   (C) Beside
   (D) Equal distance to

23

Death and Dying

1. Discuss the stages of grief

True or False

1. _____ A terminal illness will eventually cause death.

2. _____ Older people or those with terminal illnesses rarely have time to prepare for death.

3. _____ Preparing for death is a process that affects the dying person's emotions and behavior.

4. _____ All people with terminal illnesses will pass through all of the five stages described by Dr. Kubler-Ross.

5. _____ Residents may move back and forth between the stages of the process.

Multiple Choice
Read each scenario below and choose which stage the person described is in.

6. Mr. Cane was told two years ago that a tumor in his brain was inoperable and would eventually be fatal. In that time, he has visited many specialists. Despite receiving the same diagnosis from every doctor, he continues to seek further opinions, insisting that each doctor try to remove the tumor. Which stage is Mr. Cane in?
   (A) Denial
   (B) Anger
   (C) Bargaining
   (D) Depression
   (E) Acceptance

7. Mrs. Tyler is dying of heart disease. One day as her nursing assistant, Annie, is assisting her with personal care, Mrs. Tyler lashes out at her. She tells Annie that she is a dumb girl who is wasting her life and does not deserve the many years she has left to live. Which stage is Mrs. Tyler in?
   (A) Denial
   (B) Anger
   (C) Bargaining
   (D) Depression
   (E) Acceptance

8. Mr. Lopez is dying of AIDS. He has called all of his friends to say goodbye and has discussed at length with his family the kind of memorial service he would like them to arrange. What stage is Mr. Lopez in?
   (A) Denial
   (B) Anger
   (C) Bargaining
   (D) Depression
   (E) Acceptance

9. Ms. Corke has always been lively and happy. Since she has discovered that she has Lou Gehrig's disease, however, her mood has changed drastically. Although she is still healthy enough to do activities, she rarely leaves her room or even changes out of her night clothes. Which stage is Ms. Corke in?
   (A) Denial
   (B) Anger
   (C) Bargaining
   (D) Depression
   (E) Acceptance

10. Mrs. Palmer has terminal cancer. When her children try to talk to her about what kind of arrangements she wants to make for finances and her funeral, she seems not to know what they are talking about. She talks about making plans to take her granddaughter, a sophomore in high school, on a trip to Europe after her graduation. Which stage is Mrs. Palmer in?
(A) Denial
(B) Anger
(C) Bargaining
(D) Depression
(E) Acceptance

11. Mr. Celasco has had lung cancer for several years. During that time, he has tried to quit smoking but has been unsuccessful. When he finds out that there are no further treatments for him to try, he pledges that he will give up smoking in exchange for a few more years of life. What stage is Mr. Celasco in?
(A) Denial
(B) Anger
(C) Bargaining
(D) Depression
(E) Acceptance

12. Mr. Jansen suffers from Alzheimer's disease. He knows that eventually he will die from the disease and that, before then, he will become incapable of making decisions regarding his estate. He contacts his lawyer to arrange things while he still has time to make competent decisions himself. Which stage is Mr. Jansen in?
(A) Denial
(B) Anger
(C) Bargaining
(D) Depression
(E) Acceptance

2. Describe the grief process

Multiple Choice
Read each scenario below and choose which reaction to a loved one's death the person described is experiencing.

1. Malcolm's wife died during the birth of their second daughter. Malcolm is so upset with her for abandoning him and the children that he cannot even stand to hear her name spoken. What reaction is Malcolm experiencing?
(A) Loneliness
(B) Denial
(C) Anger
(D) Guilt
(E) Sadness

2. Becky's mother had been ill for many years before she died when Becky was 15. After her death, Becky remembers how she used to resent helping her mother around the house so much and wishes that she had been kinder and more cheerful. Which reaction is she having?
(A) Anger
(B) Sadness
(C) Guilt
(D) Denial
(E) Regret

3. Melinda's grandmother, to whom she was very close, died of a long illness on Sunday afternoon. On Monday morning, Melinda's mother is astonished to find Melinda getting ready for school as she does on every Monday morning. Which reaction is Melinda having?
(A) Loneliness
(B) Denial
(C) Anger
(D) Guilt
(E) Regret

4. Micah's best friend, Lawrence, died of cancer at the age of 45. Whenever Micah spends time with the friends that they had in common, he is reminded of Lawrence and feels sad. He is not as close to his other friends as he was to Lawrence, and he feels he has no one to confide in with Lawrence gone. Which reaction is he having?
(A) Shock
(B) Denial
(C) Anger
(D) Loneliness
(E) Guilt

5. Theresa's 9-year-old son went to a pool party for a friend's birthday and accidentally drowned. Theresa has been unable to forgive herself for letting him go to the party. What reaction is she having?
   (A) Anger
   (B) Loneliness
   (C) Denial
   (D) Guilt
   (E) Shock

6. Casey's brother was killed suddenly in a car accident. He is surprised that he seems to feel very little emotion regarding the death. Which reaction is Casey having?
   (A) Denial
   (B) Shock
   (C) Guilt
   (D) Anger
   (E) Regret

7. When Elizabeth's boyfriend was killed by a drunk driver on his way home one night, Elizabeth was inconsolable. She has stopped seeing her friends and stays in her room crying for hours at a time. Which reaction is she having?
   (A) Anger
   (B) Sadness
   (C) Guilt
   (D) Denial
   (E) Regret

3. Discuss how feelings and attitudes about death differ

Short Answer

1. Have you ever experienced the death of a loved one? If so, what are some of the emotions you felt?

   _____

   _____

   _____

   _____

   _____

   _____

_____

_____

_____

2. What, if any, religious or spiritual beliefs do you subscribe to? How do they influence your feelings about death? If you do not have any religious or spiritual beliefs, what are your feelings about death?

   _____

   _____

   _____

   _____

   _____

   _____

   _____

   _____

   _____

3. What cultural background do you have? What cultures are you familiar with? Briefly describe how your culture or other cultures feel about death.

   _____

   _____

   _____

   _____

   _____

   _____

   _____

   _____

   _____

   _____

142

4. Discuss how to care for a dying resident

Word Search
Fill in the blanks below and find your answers in the word search.

1. _____
   perspiring residents often; skin should be clean and dry.

2. Residents may not be able to communicate that they are in

   _____.

   Observe for signs and report them.

3. Changes of position, back massage, skin care, mouth care, and proper body

   _____

   may help to relieve pain.

4. _____
   may be one of the most important things you can do for a resident who is dying. Pay attention to these conversations.

5. _____
   can be very important. Holding your resident's hand can be comforting.

6. Do not

   _____

   the dying person or his or her family. Do not deny that death is approaching, and do not tell the resident that anyone knows how or when it will happen.

7. _____
   is usually the last sense to leave the body.

8. Give

   _____

   for visits from clergy, family, and friends.

9. Do not discuss your personal

   _____

   or spiritual beliefs with residents or their families or make recommendations.

```
x  l  t  s  r  b  l  k  j  f  d  i  n  h
v  x  v  k  a  l  i  g  n  m  e  n  t  s
r  p  c  t  s  h  s  u  n  s  t  r  o  o
x  y  w  p  z  n  t  i  h  i  b  a  u  y
x  k  e  k  r  o  e  x  b  k  r  u  c  h
y  t  r  w  m  h  n  n  o  e  e  a  h  d
b  t  j  o  t  e  i  n  l  n  v  a  e  z
a  w  k  a  s  m  n  i  v  i  u  a  o  h
w  b  b  e  g  p  g  a  r  t  u  m  s  a
k  n  a  v  o  i  d  p  f  d  j  e  y  b
t  z  b  j  o  v  v  h  l  q  o  w  t  u
e  e  p  u  l  x  g  x  v  x  a  n  r  u
f  i  s  c  c  a  g  q  v  s  u  s  v  m
k  z  s  y  w  j  q  i  t  a  w  e  o  s
```

5. Describe ways to treat dying residents and their families with dignity and honor their rights

Short Answer

1. List three legal rights to remember when working with residents who are dying.

   _____

   _____

   _____

   _____

   _____

   _____

   _____

   _____

   _____

2. Look at "The Dying Person's Bill of Rights" on pages 400-401 of your textbook. Pick three rights that you feel would be most important to you personally. Briefly describe why they would be important to you.

_____

_____

_____

_____

_____

_____

_____

_____

_____

_____

_____

_____

_____

6. Define the goals of a hospice program

Multiple Choice

1. "Hospice" is the term for compassionate care given to
   (A) Cancer patients
   (B) Dying residents
   (C) Residents with Parkinson's disease
   (D) Residents with developmental disabilities

2. Hospice care encourages the resident to
   (A) Allow hospice care teams to handle all care decisions
   (B) Allow lawyers to make care decisions
   (C) Allow doctors to make care decisions
   (D) Participate in their own care as much as possible

3. Hospice goals focus on
   (A) Recovery of the dying person
   (B) Comfort and dignity of the dying person
   (C) Curing disease
   (D) Creating a will and other legal documents for the dying person

4. Focusing on pain relief, comfort, and dignity is called _____ care.
   (A) Palliative
   (B) Personal
   (C) Professional
   (D) Pediatric

Short Answer

5. List seven attitudes and skills that are helpful in hospice care and one way you can demonstrate each.

_____

_____

_____

_____

_____

_____

_____

_____

_____

_____

_____

_____

_____

_____

_____

_____

_____

_____

_____

Name: _____

7. Explain common signs of approaching death

Short Answer

Mark an "X" next to the signs of approaching death.

1. _____ Abundance of physical activity

2. _____ Body temperature that is above or below normal

3. _____ Cold, pale skin

4. _____ Disorientation

5. _____ Healthy skin tone

6. _____ Heightened sense of touch

7. _____ Impaired speech

8. _____ Incontinence

9. _____ Perspiration

10. _____ Strong pulse

8. List changes that may occur in the human body after death

True or False

1. _____ When death occurs, the body will not have heartbeat, pulse, respiration, or blood pressure.

2. _____ The eyelids will automatically close after death.

3. _____ The body may be incontinent of both urine and stool after death.

4. _____ The muscles in the body become loose and relaxed after death.

5. _____ The nurse should be called immediately to confirm death.

9. Describe postmortem care

True or False

1. _____ The family should not be allowed to stay with the body after death.

2. _____ The body should be bathed gently to avoid bruising.

3. _____ Drainage pads are most often placed under the head and/or under the perineum.

4. _____ Remove any tubes you see coming from the body.

5. _____ Dentures should be removed from the mouth.

6. _____ You should close the eyes carefully.

7. _____ The arms should be placed on each side of the body.

8. _____ Always have a witness if any personal items are removed or given to a family member.

9. _____ After a resident has died, keep talking to the family and friends who are present so that there is no uncomfortable period of silence.

24

Caring for Your Career and Yourself

1. Discuss different types of careers in the healthcare field

True or False

1. _____ Direct service workers include salespeople, waiters, and bartenders.

2. _____ X-ray technicians work in diagnostic services.

3. _____ Receptionists, office managers, and billing staff are considered part of the healthcare field.

4. _____ Health educators have job opportunities within the healthcare field.

5. _____ Counselors and social workers are not part of the healthcare field.

2. Explain how to find a job and how to write a résumé

True or False

1. _____ The Internet is one good resource to use to try to find a job.

2. _____ If a potential employer asks for proof of your legal status in this country, it means that the employer is being discriminatory.

3. _____ Friends and relatives are the best references to use for a potential job.

4. _____ Your résumé should fit on one page.

5. _____ Your résumé should include a list of your educational experience.

6. _____ Your résumé should include a list of your religious and political beliefs.

7. _____ Your cover letter should emphasize the skills you have that would make you a good match for the position you seek.

3. Identify information that may be required when filling out a job application

Short Answer
Complete the sample job application.

Employment Application	
Personal Information	
Name:	Date:
Social Security Number:	
Home Address:	
City, State, Zip:	
Home Phone:	Business Phone:
US Citizen?	If Not, Give Visa No. and Expiration Date:

Position Applying For	
Title	Salary Desired:
Referred By:	Date Available:

Education	
High School (Name, City, State):	
Graduation Date:	
Technical or Undergraduate School:	
Dates Attended:	Degree Major:

References

146

Name: _____

4. Discuss proper job interview techniques

Short Answer
Write "Yes" or "No" next to each description below to indicate whether or not it is appropriate for a job interview.

1. _____ Arrive a couple of minutes late for the interview

2. _____ Look happy to be there

3. _____ Ask, "Do you mind if I smoke?"

4. _____ Wear very little jewelry

5. _____ Ask, "How many hours would I work?"

6. _____ Bring your child with you when you cannot find a babysitter

7. _____ Say, "I won't work with patients with AIDS."

8. _____ Sit up straight

9. _____ Ask, "What benefits do I receive with this job?"

10. _____ Shake hands with interviewer

11. _____ Eat a granola bar during the interview

12. _____ Ask, "Did I get the job?"

5. Describe a standard job description

Short Answer

1. What is a job description?

_____

_____

_____

_____

2. How does it protect employers and employees?

_____

_____

_____

_____

6. Discuss how to manage and resolve conflict

Multiple Choice

1. When is an appropriate time to discuss an issue that is causing conflict in the workplace?
   (A) When you decide you cannot take it anymore
   (B) When you are angry because something has just occurred
   (C) Right before you give your notice
   (D) When the supervisor has decided on a proper time and place

2. When trying to resolve a conflict, you should
   (A) Interrupt the other person if you might forget what you are going to say
   (B) Sit back in the chair with your arms crossed over your chest
   (C) Take turns speaking
   (D) Yell at the other person if it seems like your point is not understood

3. When discussing conflict,
   (A) State how you feel when a behavior occurs
   (B) Name-call
   (C) Don't look the other person in the eye
   (D) Keep the TV on to fill awkward silences

4. To resolve a conflict, be prepared to
   (A) Compromise
   (B) Quit
   (C) Yell
   (D) Interrupt

7. Describe employee evaluations and discuss appropriate responses to criticism

Short Answer
Read the following and mark whether they are examples of hostile or constructive criticism. Use an "H" for hostile and a "C" for constructive.

1. _____ "You are a horrible person."

2. _____ "If you weren't so slow, things might get done around here."

3. _____ "Some of your reports are not completed; try to be more accurate."

4. _____ "That was the worst meal I've ever eaten."

5. _____ "I'm not sure that you understood what I meant. Let me rephrase the issue."

6. _____ "Where did you learn how to clean?"

7. _____ "That was a stupid idea."

8. _____ "That procedure could have been performed in a more efficient way."

9. _____ "Try to make more of an effort to listen carefully."

10. _____ "Stop being so lazy."

8. Explain how to make job changes

Fill in the Blank

1. You should always give your employer

_____

weeks written notice that you will be leaving.

2. Potential future employers may talk with your past _____.

3. If you decide to change jobs, be

_____.

9. Discuss certification and explain the state's registry

Multiple Choice

1. OBRA requires that nursing assistants complete at least ___ hours of initial training before being employed.
   (A) 30
   (B) 50
   (C) 75
   (D) 100

2. OBRA requires that nursing assistants complete _____ hours of annual continuing education.
   (A) 12
   (B) 62
   (C) 75
   (D) 19

3. After completing a training course, nursing assistants are given a(n) _____ in order to be certified to work in a particular state.
   (A) Thesis
   (B) Residency
   (C) Competency exam
   (D) Apprenticeship

4. Information in each state's registry of nursing assistants includes
   (A) Personal preferences for grooming
   (B) Any findings of abuse or neglect
   (C) Mortgage information
   (D) Special diet requests

5. Moving nursing assistant certification from one state to another state is called
   (A) Call-back
   (B) Free trade
   (C) Interstate agreement
   (D) Reciprocity

10. Describe continuing education

True or False

1. _____ The federal government requires 20 hours of continuing education each year.

2. _____ Treatments or regulations can change.

3. _____ States require less continuing education than the federal government.

4. _____ In-service continuing education courses help you keep your knowledge fresh.

11. Define "stress" and "stressors"

Short Answer

What are some things that make you experience stress? How do you react when you are stressed?

_____

_____

_____

_____

_____

148

Name: _____

_____
_____
_____
_____
_____
_____
_____
_____
_____
_____
_____

12. Explain ways to manage stress

Multiple Choice

1. Stress is a _____ response.
   (A) Relaxation
   (B) Physical and emotional
   (C) Rare
   (d) Supervisory

2. When your heart beats fast in stressful situations, it can be a result of the increase of the hormone
   (A) Testosterone
   (B) Estrogen
   (C) Adrenaline
   (D) Progesterone

3. Which of the following is a physical result of the effects of stress?
   (A) Increase in heart rate
   (B) Increase in relaxation
   (C) Decrease in respiratory rate
   (D) Decrease in nervous system response

4. A healthy lifestyle is the result of
   (A) Eating when you are not hungry
   (B) Exercising regularly
   (C) Smoking a few cigarettes a week
   (D) Complaining about your job

5. Which of the following is a sign that you are not managing stress?
   (A) Preparing meals ahead of time
   (B) Taking deep breaths and relaxing
   (C) Feeling alert and positive
   (D) Not being able to focus on your work

Short Answer

6. List four places and/or people to whom you can turn to help you manage stress.

_____
_____
_____
_____
_____
_____

13. Describe a relaxation technique

Short Answer

1. Try the body scan exercise on page 413 in your textbook. Describe how you felt after the experience.

_____
_____
_____
_____
_____
_____
_____
_____
_____

2. List six things that you have done in the last month that you are happy about or proud of.

_____
_____
_____
_____
_____
_____
_____
_____
_____

14. List ways to remind yourself of the importance of the work you have chosen to do

Short Answer

1. List five things that you have learned in this course that have surprised or excited you.

_____
_____
_____
_____
_____
_____
_____
_____
_____
_____

_____
_____
_____
_____
_____
_____

2. List five things that you are looking forward to doing when you start working as a nursing assistant.

_____
_____
_____
_____
_____
_____
_____
_____
_____
_____
_____
_____
_____
_____
_____
_____
_____

Procedure Checklists

5

Preventing Infection

Washing hands			
	Procedure Steps	yes	no
1.	Turns on water at sink, keeping clothes dry.		
2.	Angles arms down, holding hands lower than elbows. Wets hands and wrists thoroughly.		
3.	Applies soap to hands.		
4.	Lathers all surfaces of hands, wrists, and fingers, producing friction, for at least 20 seconds.		
5.	Cleans nails by rubbing them in palm of other hand.		
6.	Rinses all surfaces of wrists, hands, and fingers, keeping hands lower than the elbows and the fingertips down.		
7.	Uses clean, dry paper towel to dry all surfaces of hands, wrists, and fingers. Disposes of towel without touching wastebasket.		
8.	Uses clean, dry paper towel to turn off faucet, without contaminating hands.		
9.	Disposes of used paper towel(s) in wastebasket immediately after shutting off faucet.		

_____ _____
Date Reviewed   Instructor Signature

_____ _____
Date Performed   Instructor Signature

Putting on gloves			
	Procedure Steps	yes	no
1.	Washes hands.		

2.	If right-handed, slides one glove on left hand (reverse, if left-handed).		
3.	With gloved hand, slides other hand into second glove.		
4.	Interlaces fingers to smooth out folds and create a comfortable fit.		
5.	Carefully looks for tears, holes, or spots. Replaces glove if necessary.		
6.	If wearing a gown, pulls the cuff of the gloves over the sleeve of gown.		

_____ _____
Date Reviewed   Instructor Signature

_____ _____
Date Performed   Instructor Signature

Taking off gloves			
	Procedure Steps	yes	no
1.	Touches only the outside of one glove and pulls the first glove off, turning it inside out.		
2.	With ungloved hand, reaches two fingers inside the remaining glove, without touching any part of the outside.		
3.	Pulls down, turning this glove inside out and over the first glove.		
4.	Disposes of gloves properly.		
5.	Washes hands.		

_____ _____
Date Reviewed   Instructor Signature

_____ _____
Date Performed   Instructor Signature

Name: _____

Putting on a gown

	Procedure Steps	yes	no
1.	Washes hands.		
2.	Opens gown without shaking it. Slips arms into the sleeves and pulls gown on.		
3.	Ties neck ties.		
4.	Pulls gown until it completely covers clothing. Ties the back ties.		

_____   _____
Date Reviewed   Instructor Signature

_____   _____
Date Performed   Instructor Signature

Putting on mask and goggles

	Procedure Steps	yes	no
1.	Washes hands.		
2.	Picks up mask by top strings or elastic strap. Does not touch mask where it touches face.		
3.	Adjusts mask over nose and mouth. Ties top strings first, then bottom strings.		
4.	Puts on goggles.		

_____   _____
Date Reviewed   Instructor Signature

_____   _____
Date Performed   Instructor Signature

7
Emergency Care and Disaster Preparation

Performing abdominal thrusts for the conscious person

	Procedure Steps	yes	no
1.	Obtains consent to treat the victim.		

		yes	no
2.	Stands to one side of person, putting one arm under person's arm and reaches across chest to opposite shoulder.		
3.	With other forearm and heel of hand, gives 5 sharp, separate blows to the back, between the person's shoulder blades (back blows).		
4.	If object does not come out, stands behind person and brings arms under person's arms. Wraps arms around person's waist.		
5.	Makes a fist with one hand. Places flat, thumb side of the fist against person's abdomen, above the navel but below the breastbone.		
6.	Grasps the fist with other hand. Pulls both hands toward self and up, quickly and forcefully.		
7.	Repeats 5 times, then alternates 5 back blows and 5 abdominal thrusts until object is pushed out or person loses consciousness.		
8.	Reports and documents incident.		

_____   _____
Date Reviewed   Instructor Signature

_____   _____
Date Performed   Instructor Signature

Responding to shock

	Procedure Steps	yes	no
1.	Has the person lie down on her back unless bleeding from the mouth or vomiting.		
2.	Controls bleeding if bleeding occurs.		
3.	Checks pulse and respirations if possible.		

		yes	no
4.	Keeps person as calm and comfortable as possible.		
5.	Maintains normal body temperature.		
6.	Elevates the feet unless person has a head or abdominal injury, breathing difficulties, or a fractured bone or back.		
7.	Does not give person anything to eat or drink.		
8.	Calls for help immediately.		
9.	Reports and documents incident.		

_____   _____
Date Reviewed   Instructor Signature

_____   _____
Date Performed   Instructor Signature

Responding to a heart attack

	Procedure Steps	yes	no
1.	Calls or has someone call the nurse.		
2.	Places person in a comfortable position. Encourages him to rest, and reassures him that he will not be left alone.		
3.	Loosens clothing around the neck.		
4.	Does not give person liquids or food.		
5.	Monitors person's breathing and pulse. If breathing stops or person has no pulse, performs CPR if trained to do so.		
6.	Stays with person until help arrives.		
7.	Reports and documents incident.		

_____   _____
Date Reviewed   Instructor Signature

_____   _____
Date Performed   Instructor Signature

Controlling bleeding

	Procedure Steps	yes	no
1.	Puts on gloves.		
2.	Holds thick sterile pad, clean pad, or a clean cloth against the wound.		
3.	Presses down hard directly on the bleeding wound until help arrives. Does not decrease pressure. Puts additional pads over the first pad if blood seeps through. Does not remove the first pad.		
4.	Raises the wound above the level of the heart to slow down the bleeding.		
5.	When bleeding is under control, secures the dressing to keep it in place. Checks person for symptoms of shock. Stays with person until help arrives.		
6.	Removes gloves and washes hands.		
7.	Reports and documents incident.		

_____   _____
Date Reviewed   Instructor Signature

_____   _____
Date Performed   Instructor Signature

Responding to poisoning

	Procedure Steps	yes	no
1.	Notifies nurse immediately.		
2.	Looks for a container that will help determine what the resident has taken or eaten. Using gloves, checks the mouth for chemical burns and notes breath odor.		
3.	Follows instructions from poison control center if asked to call.		

4.	Reports and documents incident.		

Date Reviewed	Instructor Signature

Date Performed	Instructor Signature

8.	Reports and documents incident.		

Date Reviewed	Instructor Signature

Date Performed	Instructor Signature

Treating burns

	Procedure Steps	yes	no
	Minor burns:		
1.	Uses cool, clean water (not ice) to decrease the skin temperature and prevent further injury (does not use ointment, salve, or grease).		
2.	Dampens a clean cloth and covers burn.		
3.	Covers area with dry, sterile gauze.		
	Serious burns:		
1.	Removes person from the source of burn.		
2.	Calls for emergency help.		
3.	Checks for breathing, pulse, and severe bleeding. Does not apply water.		
4.	Does not remove clothing from burned areas. Covers burn with thick, dry, sterile gauze or a clean cloth (does not apply water or use ointment, salve, or grease).		
5.	Elevates affected part after person lies down.		
6.	If the burn covers a larger area, wraps person in a dry, clean sheet. Takes care not to rub the skin.		
7.	Waits for emergency medical help.		

Responding to fainting

	Procedure Steps	yes	no
1.	Has person lie down or sit down before fainting occurs.		
2.	If person is in a sitting position, has her bend forward and place her head between her knees. If person is lying flat on her back, elevates the legs.		
3.	Loosens any tight clothing.		
4.	Has person stay in position for at least five minutes after symptoms disappear.		
5.	Helps person get up slowly. Continues to observe her for symptoms of fainting.		
6.	Reports and documents incident.		

Date Reviewed	Instructor Signature

Date Performed	Instructor Signature

Responding to a nosebleed

	Procedure Steps	yes	no
1.	Elevates head of the bed or tells person to remain in sitting position. Offers tissues or a clean cloth.		
2.	Puts on gloves. Applies firm pressure over the bridge of the nose. Squeezes bridge of nose with thumb and forefinger.		
3.	Applies pressure consistently until bleeding stops.		

4.	Uses a cool cloth or ice wrapped in a cloth on back of neck, forehead, or upper lip to slow blood flow. Tells nurse immediately if bleeding does not stop.		
5.	Reports and documents incident.		

_____ _____
Date Reviewed   Instructor Signature

_____ _____
Date Performed   Instructor Signature

Responding to seizures

	Procedure Steps	yes	no
1.	Lowers person to the floor and lays him on his side.		
2.	Has someone call nurse immediately or uses call light. Does not leave person unless has to get medical help.		
3.	Moves furniture away to prevent injury. If a pillow is nearby, places it under his head.		
4.	Does not try to restrain the person.		
5.	Does not force anything between the person's teeth. Does not place hands in person's mouth.		
6.	Does not give liquids or food.		
7.	When the seizure is over, checks breathing.		
8.	Reports and documents incident.		

_____ _____
Date Reviewed   Instructor Signature

_____ _____
Date Performed   Instructor Signature

Responding to vomiting

	Procedure Steps	yes	no
1.	Puts on gloves.		
2.	Provides a basin and removes it when vomiting has stopped.		
3.	Removes soiled linens or clothes and replaces with fresh ones.		
4.	Measures and notes amount of vomitus, if monitoring resident's I&O.		
5.	Discards vomit in toilet unless vomit is red, has blood in it, or looks like coffee grounds. Washes and stores basin properly.		
6.	Removes and discards gloves.		
7.	Washes hands.		
8.	Puts on fresh gloves.		
9.	Provides comfort to resident.		
10.	Puts soiled linens in proper container.		
11.	Removes and discards gloves.		
12.	Washes hands again.		
13.	Documents time, amount, color, and consistency of vomitus.		

_____ _____
Date Reviewed   Instructor Signature

_____ _____
Date Performed   Instructor Signature

10
Positioning, Lifting, and Moving

Helping a resident sit up using the arm lock

	Procedure Steps	yes	no
1.	Washes hands.		
2.	Identifies self by name. Identifies resident by name.		
3.	Explains procedure to resident, speaking clearly, slowly, and directly. Maintains face-to-face contact whenever possible.		

Name: _____

		yes	no
4.	Provides privacy.		
5.	Adjusts the bed to safe working level, usually waist high. Locks bed wheels.		
6.	Stands facing the bed with legs about 12 inches apart and knees bent. Puts foot farther from the bed slightly ahead of the other foot.		
7.	Places arm under resident's armpit and grasps resident's shoulder, while resident grasps caregiver's shoulder.		
8.	Reaches under resident's head and places other hand on resident's far shoulder. Has resident bend knees. Bends own knees.		
9.	Rocks backward at the count of three and pulls resident to sitting position.		
10.	Observes resident for dizziness or weakness.		
11.	Returns bed to lowest position.		
12.	Places call light within resident's reach.		
13.	Washes hands.		
14.	Documents procedure.		

_____   _____
Date Reviewed   Instructor Signature

_____   _____
Date Performed   Instructor Signature

Moving a resident up in bed			
	Procedure Steps	yes	no
If resident can assist:			
1.	Washes hands.		
2.	Identifies self by name. Identifies resident by name.		
3.	Explains procedure to resident, speaking clearly, slowly, and directly. Maintains face-to-face contact whenever possible.		

		yes	no
4.	Provides privacy.		
5.	Adjusts the bed to safe working level, usually waist high. Locks bed wheels. Lowers head of bed to make it flat. Removes the pillow and places it at head of bed standing upright.		
6.	Raises side rail on far side of bed.		
7.	Stands by bed with feet apart, facing resident. Places one arm under resident's shoulders and the other under resident's thighs.		
8.	Instructs resident to bend knees, brace feet on mattress, and push down with her feet and hands on the count of three.		
9.	On count, shifts body weight and helps resident to move toward the head of the bed while she pushes with her feet.		
10.	Positions resident comfortably, arranges pillow and blankets, and returns bed to lowest position.		
11.	Places call light within resident's reach.		
12.	Washes hands.		
13.	Documents procedure.		

_____   _____
Date Reviewed   Instructor Signature

_____   _____
Date Performed   Instructor Signature

		yes	no
If resident cannot assist:			
1.	Follows steps 1 through 5 above.		
2.	Stands behind head of bed with feet apart and one foot slightly in front of other.		
3.	Rolls and grasps top of draw sheet, bends knees, keeping back straight, and rocks weight from front foot to back foot.		

4.	Positions resident comfortably, arranges pillow and blankets, unrolls draw sheet, and returns bed to lowest position.		
5.	Places call light within resident's reach.		
6.	Washes hands.		
7.	Documents procedure.		

_____   _____
Date Reviewed   Instructor Signature

_____   _____
Date Performed   Instructor Signature

	When you have help from another person and resident cannot assist:		
1.	Follows steps 1 through 5 above.		
2.	Stands on opposite side of bed from helper. Turns slightly toward the head of bed, points foot closest toward head of bed. Stands with feet apart and knees bent.		
3.	Rolls and grasps top of draw sheet with palms up.		
4.	Shifts weight to back foot and on count of three, both workers shift weight to forward feet while sliding draw sheet toward head of bed.		
5.	Positions resident comfortably, arranges pillow and blankets, unrolls draw sheet, and returns bed to lowest position.		
6.	Places call light within resident's reach.		
7.	Washes hands.		
8.	Documents procedure.		

_____   _____
Date Reviewed   Instructor Signature

_____   _____
Date Performed   Instructor Signature

Moving a resident to the side of the bed

	Procedure Steps	yes	no
1.	Washes hands.		
2.	Identifies self by name. Identifies resident by name.		
3.	Explains procedure to resident, speaking clearly, slowly, and directly. Maintains face-to-face contact whenever possible.		
4.	Provides privacy.		
5.	Adjusts the bed to safe working level, usually waist high. Locks bed wheels. Lowers head of bed.		
6.	Stands on same side of bed to where resident will be moved.		
7.	**With a draw sheet:** Rolls draw sheet up and grasps draw sheet with palms up. Puts hand at resident's shoulders, and the other at resident's hips. Applies one knee against side of bed, leans back and pulls draw sheet and resident on the count of three.		
	Without a draw sheet: Slides hands under head and shoulders and moves toward self. Slides hands under midsection and moves toward self. Slides hands under hips and legs and moves toward self.		
8.	Returns bed to lowest position.		
9.	Places call light within resident's reach.		
10.	Washes hands.		
11.	Documents procedure.		

_____   _____
Date Reviewed   Instructor Signature

_____   _____
Date Performed   Instructor Signature

158

Turning a resident

	Procedure Steps	yes	no
1.	Washes hands.		
2.	Identifies self by name. Identifies resident by name.		
3.	Explains procedure to resident, speaking clearly, slowly, and directly. Maintains face-to-face contact whenever possible.		
4.	Provides privacy.		
5.	Adjusts the bed to a safe working level, usually waist high. Locks bed wheels. Lowers head of bed.		
6.	Stands at opposite side of the bed to where resident will be turned. Raises far side rail and lowers near side rail.		
7.	Moves resident to side of bed using proper procedure.		
	Turning resident away from you:		
8.	Crosses resident's arm over chest and moves arm on side resident is being turned to out of the way. Crosses leg nearest self over far leg. Stands with feet about 12 inches apart, bends knees, and places one hand on resident's shoulder and the other on the nearest hip. Pushes resident toward other side of bed while shifting weight from back leg to front leg.		
	Turning resident toward you:		
8.	Crosses resident's arm over chest and moves arm on side resident is being turned to out of the way. Crosses leg farthest from self over near leg. Stands with feet about 12 inches apart, bends knees and places one hand on resident's far shoulder and the other on the far hip. Rolls resident toward self.		

		yes	no
9.	Positions resident comfortably using pillows or other supports, and checks for good alignment.		
10.	Returns bed to lowest position.		
11.	Places call light within resident's reach.		
12.	Washes hands.		
13.	Documents procedure.		

_____   _____
Date Reviewed   Instructor Signature

_____   _____
Date Performed   Instructor Signature

Logrolling a resident with one assistant

	Procedure Steps	yes	no
1.	Washes hands.		
2.	Identifies self by name. Identifies resident by name.		
3.	Explains procedure to resident, speaking clearly, slowly, and directly. Maintains face-to-face contact whenever possible.		
4.	Provides privacy.		
5.	Adjusts the bed to safe working level, usually waist high. Locks bed wheels. Lowers head of bed to make it flat. Lowers side rail on side closest to self.		
6.	Both workers stand on same side of bed, one at the resident's head and shoulders, one near the midsection.		
7.	Places resident's arm across his chest and places pillow between the knees.		
8.	Stands with feet about 12 inches apart, bends knees, and grasps draw sheet on far side.		
9.	Rolls resident toward self on count of three, turning resident as a unit.		
10.	Positions resident comfortably with pillows or supports, and checks for good alignment.		

		yes	no
11.	Returns bed to lowest position.		
12.	Places call light within resident's reach.		
13.	Washes hands.		
14.	Documents procedure.		

_____ _____
Date Reviewed   Instructor Signature

_____ _____
Date Performed   Instructor Signature

Assisting a resident to sit up on side of bed: dangling			
	Procedure Steps	yes	no
1.	Washes hands.		
2.	Identifies self by name. Identifies resident by name.		
3.	Explains procedure to resident, speaking clearly, slowly, and directly. Maintains face-to-face contact whenever possible.		
4.	Provides privacy.		
5.	Adjusts the bed to lowest position. Locks bed wheels.		
6.	Fanfolds top covers to foot of bed and assists resident to turn onto side, facing self.		
7.	Has resident reach across chest with top arm and place hand on edge of bed near opposite shoulder. Asks resident to push down on that hand while swinging legs over the side of bed.		
8.	If resident needs assistance, raises head of bed to sitting position. Stands with legs 12 inches apart, with one foot 6 to 8 inches in front of the other. Bends knees.		
9.	Places one arm under resident's shoulder blades and the other under her thighs.		
10.	On the count of three, turns resident into sitting position.		

		yes	no
11.	With resident holding onto edge of mattress, puts non-skid shoes on resident.		
12.	Has resident dangle as long as ordered. Does not leave resident alone.		
13.	Assists resident back into bed by placing one arm around resident's shoulders. Places other arm under resident's knees and slowly swings resident's legs onto the bed.		
14.	Leaves bed in lowest position.		
15.	Places call light within resident's reach.		
16.	Washes hands.		
17.	Documents procedure.		

_____ _____
Date Reviewed   Instructor Signature

_____ _____
Date Performed   Instructor Signature

Applying a transfer belt			
	Procedure Steps	yes	no
1.	Washes hands.		
2.	Identifies self by name. Identifies resident by name.		
3.	Explains procedure to resident, speaking clearly, slowly, and directly. Maintains face-to-face contact whenever possible.		
4.	Provides privacy.		
5.	Assists resident to sitting position.		
6.	Places the belt over the resident's clothing and around the waist. Does not put it over bare skin.		
7.	Tightens the buckle until it is snug. Leaves enough room to insert two fingers comfortably into the belt. Checks to make sure that a female's breasts are not caught under the belt.		

8.	For comfort, places the buckle off-center in the front or back.		

_____ _____
Date Reviewed   Instructor Signature

_____ _____
Date Performed   Instructor Signature

Transferring a resident from bed to wheelchair

	Procedure Steps	yes	no
1.	Washes hands.		
2.	Identifies self by name. Identifies resident by name.		
3.	Explains procedure to resident, speaking clearly, slowly, and directly. Maintains face-to-face contact whenever possible.		
4.	Provides privacy.		
5.	Removes footrests close to the bed and places chair near the head of the bed on resident's stronger side. Locks wheelchair wheels.		
6.	Raises head of bed and adjusts bed level so that the height of bed is equal to or slightly higher than chair. Locks bed wheels.		
7.	Assists resident to sitting position with feet flat on floor. Puts non-skid shoes on resident and fastens.		
8.	**With transfer belt:** Stands in front of resident with feet about 12 inches apart. Bends knees. Places transfer belt around resident's waist and grasps belt on both sides.		
	Without transfer belt: Stands in front of resident with feet about 12 inches apart. Bends knees. Places arms around resident's torso under her arms and asks resident to use the bed to push up.		

9.	Provides instructions to assist with transfer. Braces legs against resident's lower legs. Helps resident stand on count of three.		
10.	Instructs resident to take small steps to the chair while turning back toward chair. Assists resident to pivot to front of chair if necessary.		
11.	Asks resident to put hands on chair arm rests and helps resident to lower herself into the chair when chair is touching back of resident's legs.		
12.	Repositions resident with hips touching back of wheelchair. Removes transfer belt and attaches footrests and places resident's feet on them. Positions resident comfortably, checking for good alignment and placing robe or blanket over lap.		
13.	Places call light within resident's reach.		
14.	Washes hands.		
15.	Documents procedure.		

_____ _____
Date Reviewed   Instructor Signature

_____ _____
Date Performed   Instructor Signature

Transferring a resident from bed to stretcher

	Procedure Steps	yes	no
1.	Washes hands.		
2.	Identifies self by name. Identifies resident by name.		
3.	Explains procedure to resident. Speaks clearly, slowly, and directly. Maintains face-to-face contact whenever possible.		
4.	Provides privacy.		
5.	Lowers head of bed so that it is flat. Locks bed wheels.		

Name: _____ 161

		yes	no
6.	Lowers side rail on side to which resident will be moved.		
7.	Moves resident to side of bed.		
8.	Lowers side rail on other side of bed, keeping a hand on resident at all times.		
9.	Places stretcher against bed with height of bed equal to height of stretcher. Locks stretcher wheels. Removes safety belts.		
10.	Two workers stand on one side of resident, while two others stand behind the stretcher. Each worker rolls up sides of draw sheet.		
11.	On count of three, workers lift and move resident to stretcher, centering him or her.		
12.	Places pillow under resident's head and covers resident. Places safety straps across resident and raises side rails on stretcher.		
13.	Unlocks stretcher's wheels. Takes resident to proper place, staying with resident until another staff member takes over.		
14.	Washes hands.		
15.	Documents procedure.		

_____   _____
Date Reviewed   Instructor Signature

_____   _____
Date Performed   Instructor Signature

Transferring a resident using a mechanical lift

	Procedure Steps	yes	no
1.	Washes hands.		
2.	Identifies self by name. Identifies resident by name.		
3.	Explains procedure to resident, speaking clearly, slowly, and directly. Maintains face-to-face contact whenever possible.		
4.	Provides privacy.		
5.	Locks bed wheels. Positions wheelchair next to bed and locks brakes.		
6.	With resident turned to one side of bed, positions sling under resident. Helps resident roll back to middle of bed and spreads out fanfolded edge of sling.		
7.	Positions mechanical lift next to bed, opening the base to its widest point, and pushes base of lift under bed. Positions overhead bar directly over resident.		
8.	Attaches straps to sling properly.		
9.	Raises resident in sling two inches above bed, following manufacturer's instructions. Pauses for resident to gain balance.		
10.	Rolls mechanical lift to position resident over chair or wheelchair. Lifting partner supports and guides resident's body.		
11.	Slowly lowers resident into chair or wheelchair, pushing down gently on resident's knees.		
12.	Undoes straps from overhead bar to sling, leaving sling in place.		
13.	Positions resident comfortably, checking for good alignment.		
14.	Places call light within resident's reach.		
15.	Washes hands.		
16.	Documents procedure.		

_____   _____
Date Reviewed   Instructor Signature

_____   _____
Date Performed   Instructor Signature

162

Name: _____

Transferring a resident onto and off of a toilet

	Procedure Steps	yes	no
1.	Washes hands.		
2.	Identifies self by name. Identifies resident by name.		
3.	Explains procedure to resident. Speaks clearly, slowly, and directly. Maintains face-to-face contact whenever possible.		
4.	Provides privacy.		
5.	Positions wheelchair at right angle to the toilet to face hand bar.		
6.	Removes footrests. Locks wheels.		
7.	Applies a transfer belt. Grasps the belt, putting one hand toward resident's back and one toward resident's front.		
8.	Asks resident to push against armrests of wheelchair to stand, reaching for and grasping the hand bar.		
9.	Asks resident to pivot and back up to feel front of toilet with back of her legs.		
10.	Helps resident pull down underwear and pants.		
11.	Helps resident sit down slowly.		
12.	When resident is done, applies gloves. Assists with perineal care as necessary.		
13.	Cleans and dries resident. Removes and disposes of gloves. Washes hands.		
14.	Pulls up clothing. Helps with handwashing as necessary.		
15.	Helps resident into wheelchair.		
16.	Washes hands again.		
17.	Helps resident leave bathroom.		
18.	Places call light within resident's reach.		
19.	Reports any changes in resident.		
20.	Documents procedure.		

Date Reviewed _____ Instructor Signature _____

Date Performed _____ Instructor Signature _____

Transferring a resident into a car

	Procedure Steps	yes	no
1.	Washes hands.		
2.	Identifies self by name. Identifies resident by name.		
3.	Explains procedure to resident. Speaks clearly, slowly, and directly. Maintains face-to-face contact whenever possible.		
4.	Places wheelchair close to car at a 45-degree angle. Opens car door on resident's stronger side. Locks wheelchair.		
5.	Asks resident to push against armrests of wheelchair to come to a standing position.		
6.	Asks resident to grasp the car and pivot foot so that car seat touches the back of the legs.		
7.	Helps resident sit in car, lifting one leg, then the other into the car.		
8.	Positions resident comfortably and secures seat belt.		
9.	Carefully shuts door.		
10.	Returns wheelchair to proper site.		
11.	Washes hands.		
12.	Documents procedure.		

Date Reviewed _____ Instructor Signature _____

Date Performed _____ Instructor Signature _____

Assisting a resident to ambulate

	Procedure Steps	yes	no
1.	Washes hands.		
2.	Identifies self by name. Identifies resident by name.		
3.	Explains procedure to resident, speaking clearly, slowly, and directly. Maintains face-to-face contact whenever possible.		
4.	Provides privacy.		
5.	Puts non-skid footwear on resident. Adjusts the bed to low position so that feet are flat on the floor. Locks bed wheels.		
6.	Stands in front of and faces resident.		
7.	Braces resident's lower extremities and bends knees. Places one foot between resident's knees.		
8.	**With transfer belt:** Places belt around resident's waist. Bends knees, leans forward, and grasps the belt. Has resident lean forward, push down on bed with her hands, and stand on count of three. On count of three, rocks weight onto back foot to assist resident to standing position.		
	Without transfer belt: Places arms around resident's torso under armpits, while assisting resident to stand.		
9.	**With transfer belt:** Walks slightly behind and to one side of resident for distance while holding on to transfer belt.		
	Without transfer belt: Walks slightly behind and to one side of the resident for full distance, supporting resident's back with arm. Stands on weaker side.		
10.	Observes resident's strength and provides chair if resident becomes tired.		
11.	Removes transfer belt and returns the resident safely to bed or a chair. Positions resident comfortably. Returns bed to lowest position.		
12.	Places call light within resident's reach.		
13.	Washes hands.		
14.	Documents procedure.		

_____ _____
Date Reviewed   Instructor Signature

_____ _____
Date Performed   Instructor Signature

Assisting with ambulation for a resident using a cane, walker, or crutches

	Procedure Steps	yes	no
1.	Washes hands.		
2.	Identifies self by name. Identifies resident by name.		
3.	Explains procedure to resident, speaking clearly, slowly, and directly. Maintains face-to-face contact whenever possible.		
4.	Provides privacy.		
5.	Puts non-skid footwear on resident. Adjusts the bed to low position so that feet are flat on the floor. Locks bed wheels.		
6.	Stands in front of and faces resident.		
7.	Braces resident's lower extremities and bends knees. Places one foot between resident's knees.		
8.	Places gait belt around resident's waist and grasps the belt, while assisting resident to stand.		
9.	Helps as needed with ambulation with cane, walker, or crutches, walking slightly behind or on the weak side of resident.		

10.	Watches for obstacles in the resident's path.		
11.	Lets the resident set the pace, encouraging rest as necessary.		
12.	Removes gait belt. Returns the resident safely to bed or a chair and positions resident comfortably. Returns bed to lowest position.		
13.	Places call light within resident's reach.		
14.	Washes hands.		
15.	Documents procedure.		

_____   _____
Date Reviewed   Instructor Signature

_____   _____
Date Performed   Instructor Signature

	Helps resident put personal items away.		
	Provides fresh water.		
6.	Orients resident to the room and bathroom. Explains how to work equipment.		
7.	Introduces resident to roommate, other residents, and staff.		
8.	Makes resident comfortable.		
9.	Places call light within resident's reach.		
10.	Washes hands.		
11.	Documents procedure.		

_____   _____
Date Reviewed   Instructor Signature

_____   _____
Date Performed   Instructor Signature

11
Admitting, Transferring, and Discharging

Admitting a resident			
	Procedure Steps	yes	no
1.	Washes hands.		
2.	Identifies self by name. Identifies resident by name.		
3.	Explains procedure to resident. Speaks clearly, slowly, and directly. Maintains face-to-face contact whenever possible.		
4.	Provides privacy.		
5.	If part of facility procedure, performs the following:		
	Takes resident's height and weight.		
	Takes resident's baseline vital signs.		
	Obtains a urine specimen if required.		
	Completes the paperwork, including an inventory of all personal items.		

Measuring and recording weight of an ambulatory resident			
	Procedure Steps	yes	no
1.	Washes hands.		
2.	Identifies self by name. Identifies resident by name.		
3.	Explains procedure to resident. Speaks clearly, slowly, and directly. Maintains face-to-face contact whenever possible.		
4.	Provides privacy.		
5.	Starts with scale balanced at zero before weighing resident.		
6.	Helps resident to step onto the center of the scale.		
7.	Determines resident's weight.		
8.	Assists resident off scale before recording weight.		
9.	Records weight.		
10.	Places call light within resident's reach.		
11.	Washes hands.		

12.	Documents procedure.		

_____ _____
Date Reviewed   Instructor Signature

_____ _____
Date Performed   Instructor Signature

Measuring and recording height of a resident			
	Procedure Steps	yes	no
	For residents who cannot get out of bed:		
1.	Washes hands.		
2.	Identifies self by name. Identifies resident by name.		
3.	Explains procedure to resident. Speaks clearly, slowly, and directly. Maintains face-to-face contact whenever possible.		
4.	Provides privacy.		
5.	Positions resident lying straight in bed, flat on his back.		
6.	Makes a pencil mark on the sheet at the top of the head. Makes another mark at the resident's heel. Measures the distance between the marks.		
7.	Records height.		
8.	Places call light within resident's reach.		
9.	Washes hands.		
10.	Documents procedure.		

_____ _____
Date Reviewed   Instructor Signature

_____ _____
Date Performed   Instructor Signature

	For residents who can get out of bed:		
1.	Follows steps 1 through 4 above.		
2.	Helps resident to step onto scale, facing away from scale.		

3.	Asks resident to stand straight. Helps as needed.		
4.	Pulls up measuring rod from back of scale. Gently lowers measuring rod until it rests flat on resident's head.		
5.	Determines resident's height.		
6.	Helps resident off scale before recording height.		
7.	Records height.		
8.	Places call light within resident's reach.		
9.	Washes hands.		
10.	Documents procedure.		

_____ _____
Date Reviewed   Instructor Signature

_____ _____
Date Performed   Instructor Signature

Transferring a resident			
	Procedure Steps	yes	no
1.	Washes hands.		
2.	Identifies self by name. Identifies resident by name.		
3.	Explains procedure to resident. Speaks clearly, slowly, and directly. Maintains face-to-face contact whenever possible.		
4.	Provides privacy.		
5.	Collects the items to be transferred and takes them to the new location.		
6.	Assists resident into the wheelchair or stretcher. Takes him or her to proper area.		
7.	Introduces new residents and staff.		
8.	Helps resident to put personal items away.		

		yes	no
9.	Makes resident comfortable. Places call light within resident's reach.		
10.	Washes hands.		
11.	Documents procedure.		

_____   _____
Date Reviewed   Instructor Signature

_____   _____
Date Performed   Instructor Signature

Discharging a resident

	Procedure Steps	yes	no
1.	Washes hands.		
2.	Identifies self by name. Identifies resident by name.		
3.	Explains procedure to resident. Speaks clearly, slowly, and directly. Maintains face-to-face contact whenever possible.		
4.	Provides privacy.		
5.	Compares the checklist to the items there. If all items are there, asks resident to sign.		
6.	Collects the items to be taken and takes them to pickup area.		
7.	Assists resident to dress and then into the wheelchair or stretcher.		
8.	Assists resident to say good-byes to the staff and residents.		
9.	Takes resident to the pickup area. Assists resident into vehicle.		
10.	Washes hands.		
11.	Documents procedure.		

_____   _____
Date Reviewed   Instructor Signature

_____   _____
Date Performed   Instructor Signature

12
The Resident's Unit

Making an occupied bed

	Procedure Steps	yes	no
1.	Washes hands.		
2.	Identifies self by name. Identifies resident by name.		
3.	Explains procedure to resident, speaking clearly, slowly, and directly. Maintains face-to-face contact whenever possible.		
4.	Provides privacy.		
5.	Places clean linen on clean surface within reach (e.g. bedside stand, overbed table, or chair).		
6.	Adjusts the bed to a safe working level, usually waist high. Lowers head of bed. Locks bed wheels.		
7.	Puts on gloves.		
8.	Loosens top linen from working side. Unfolds bath blanket over top sheet to cover resident and removes top sheet.		
9.	Raises side rail on far side of bed and turns resident onto her side, away from self, toward raised side rail.		
10.	Loosens bottom soiled linen, mattress pad, and protector on working side.		
11.	Rolls bottom soiled linen toward resident, tucking it snugly against the resident's back.		
12.	Places and tucks in clean bottom linen, finishing with no wrinkles. Makes hospital corners if necessary.		
13.	Smoothes bottom sheet out toward the resident. Rolls extra material toward resident and tucks it under resident's body.		

14.	Places waterproof pad if using and centers it. Tucks side near self under mattress and smoothes it out toward resident.		
15.	Places draw sheet if using. Smoothes and tucks as with other bedding.		
16.	Raises side rail nearest self and lowers side rail on other side of bed. Assists resident to turn onto clean bottom sheet.		
17.	Loosens soiled linen. Rolls linen from head to the foot of bed, avoiding contact with skin or clothes. Places it in hamper or bag.		
18.	Pulls and tucks in clean bottom linen just like other side, finishing with bottom sheet free of wrinkles.		
19.	Asks resident to turn onto his or her back, keeping resident covered. Raises side rail.		
20.	Unfolds top sheet and places it over resident. Asks resident to hold onto top sheet and slips blanket or old sheet out from underneath. Puts it in hamper or bag.		
21.	Places a blanket over the top sheet, matching the top edges. Tucks bottom edges of top sheet and blanket under mattress, making hospital corners on each side. Loosens top linens over resident's feet. Folds top sheet over the blanket about six inches.		
22.	Removes pillow and pillowcase. Places it in hamper or bag. Removes gloves.		
23.	Places clean pillowcases on pillows. Places them under resident's head with open end away from door.		
24.	Returns bed to lowest position.		

25.	Places call light within resident's reach.		
26.	Takes hamper or bag to proper area.		
27.	Washes hands.		
28.	Documents procedure.		

_____   _____
Date Reviewed   Instructor Signature

_____   _____
Date Performed   Instructor Signature

Making an unoccupied bed			
	Procedure Steps	yes	no
1.	Washes hands.		
2.	Places clean linen within reach (e.g. bedside stand, overbed table, or chair).		
3.	Adjusts the bed to a safe working level, usually waist high. Puts bed in flattest position. Locks bed wheels.		
4.	Puts on gloves.		
5.	Loosens soiled linen and rolls it from head to foot of bed. Avoids contact with skin or clothes. Places it in a hamper or bag.		
6.	Removes and discards gloves. Washes hands.		
7.	Remakes bed, spreading mattress pad and bottom sheet, tucking under. Makes hospital corners. Puts on mattress protector and draw sheet, smoothes, and tucks under sides of bed.		
8.	Places top sheet and blanket, centering them. Tucks under end of bed and makes hospital corners. Folds down top sheet over the blanket about six inches.		

9.	Removes pillows and pillowcases. Puts on clean pillowcases. Replaces pillows.		
10.	Returns bed to its lowest position.		
11.	Takes hamper or bag to proper area.		
12.	Washes hands.		
13.	Documents procedure.		

_____ _____
Date Reviewed   Instructor Signature

_____ _____
Date Performed   Instructor Signature

Making a surgical bed

	Procedure Steps	yes	no
1.	Washes hands.		
2.	Places clean linen within reach.		
3.	Adjusts the bed to a safe level, usually waist high. Locks bed wheels.		
4.	Puts on gloves.		
5.	Loosens soiled linen and rolls it from head to foot of bed. Avoids contact with skin or clothes. Places it in hamper or bag.		
6.	Removes and discards gloves. Washes hands.		
7.	Makes an unoccupied, closed bed, with bedding left up.		
8.	Loosens linens on side of bed that is away from door (where stretcher will be).		
9.	Fanfolds linens lengthwise to the side away from door.		
10.	Puts on clean pillowcases. Replaces pillows.		
11.	Leaves bed in locked position with both side rails down.		
12.	Makes sure pathway to bed is clear.		

13.	Takes hamper or bag to proper area.		
14.	Washes hands.		
15.	Documents procedure.		

_____ _____
Date Reviewed   Instructor Signature

_____ _____
Date Performed   Instructor Signature

13
Personal Care Skills

Giving a complete bed bath

	Procedure Steps	yes	no
1.	Washes hands.		
2.	Identifies self by name. Identifies resident by name.		
3.	Explains procedure to resident, speaking clearly, slowly, and directly. Maintains face-to-face contact whenever possible.		
4.	Provides privacy.		
5.	Adjusts the bed to a safe working level, usually waist high. Locks bed wheels.		
6.	Places blanket over resident and removes top bedding and gown while keeping resident covered.		
7.	Fills basin and checks temperature (105°F to 110°F). Has resident test water temperature and adjusts if necessary.		
8.	Puts on gloves.		
9.	Asks and assists resident to participate in washing.		
10.	Uncovers only one part of the body at a time. Places a towel under the body part being washed.		
11.	Washes, rinses, and dries one part of the body at a time. Starts at the head, works down, and completes front first.		

	Eyes and Face: Washes face with wet washcloth (no soap) beginning with the eyes, using a different area of the washcloth for each eye, washing inner aspect to outer aspect. Washes the face from the middle outward using firm but gentle strokes. Washes neck and ears and behind the ears. Rinses and pats dry.				**Back**: Helps resident move to the center of the bed, then turns onto his side so back is facing self. Washes back, neck, and buttocks with long, downward strokes. Rinses and pats dry. Applies lotion if ordered.		
	Arms: Washes upper arm and underarm. Uses long strokes from the shoulder down to the wrist. Rinses and pats dry.			12.	Places towel under buttocks and thighs and helps resident turn onto his back. Puts on gloves if not already on.		
	Wash the hand in a basin: Cleans under nails. Rinses and pats dry. Gives nail care. Repeats for other arm and hand. Applies lotion if ordered.			13.	**Perineal area and buttocks**: Changes bath water. Washes, rinses, and dries perineal area, working from front to back.		
	Chest: Pulls blanket down to waist. Lifts the towel only enough to wash the chest, rinse it, and pat dry. For a female resident: washes, rinses, and dries breasts and under breasts.				**For a female resident**: Washes the perineum with soap and water from front to back, using single strokes. Uses a clean area of washcloth or clean washcloth for each stroke. Wipes the center of the perineum, then each side. Spreads the labia majora. Wipes from front to back on each side. Rinses the area in the same way. Dries entire perineal area moving from front to back, using a blotting motion with towel. Asks resident to turn on her side. Washes, rinses, and dries buttocks and anal area. Cleanses anal area without contaminating the perineal area.		
	Abdomen: Folds blanket down so that pubic area is still covered. Washes abdomen, rinses, and pats dry.						
	Legs and Feet: Exposes one leg and places towel under it. Washes the thigh. Uses long downward strokes. Rinses and pats dry. Does the same from the knee to the ankle. Washes the foot and between the toes in a basin. Rinses foot and pats dry, making sure area between toes is dry. Provides nail care if it has been assigned. Applies lotion if ordered but not between the toes. Repeats steps for other leg and foot.						

		yes	no
	For a male resident: If resident is uncircumcised, retracts the foreskin first. Gently pushes skin toward the base of penis. Holds the penis by the shaft and washes in a circular motion from the tip down to the base. Uses a clean area of washcloth or clean washcloth for each stroke. Rinses the penis. If resident is uncircumcised, gently returns foreskin to normal position. Then washes the scrotum and groin. Rinses and pats dry. Asks resident to turn on his side. Washes, rinses, and dries buttocks and anal area. Cleanses anal area without contaminating the perineal area.		
14.	Covers resident. Disposes of water and cleans and stores bath basin. Places soiled clothing and linens in proper container.		
15.	Removes and disposes of gloves and washes hands.		
16.	Puts clean gown on resident and assists with grooming as necessary.		
17.	Returns bed to lowest position.		
18.	Places call light within resident's reach.		
19.	Washes hands.		
20.	Documents procedure.		

_____ _____
Date Reviewed   Instructor Signature

_____ _____
Date Performed   Instructor Signature

Giving a back rub

	Procedure Steps	yes	no
1.	Washes hands.		
2.	Identifies self by name. Identifies resident by name.		
3.	Explains procedure to resident, speaking clearly, slowly, and directly. Maintains face-to-face contact whenever possible.		
4.	Provides privacy.		
5.	Adjusts the bed to safe working level, usually waist high. Lowers head of bed. Locks bed wheels.		
6.	Positions resident in prone position or side position. Covers resident with blanket and folds back bed covers, exposing resident's back to the top of the buttocks.		
7.	Warms lotion and hands. Pours lotion onto hands and rubs hands together.		
8.	Starting at the upper part of the buttocks, makes long, smooth upward strokes with both hands. Circles hands up along spine, shoulders, and then back down along the outer edges of the back. At buttocks, makes another circle back up to the shoulders. Repeats for three to five minutes.		
9.	Starting at the base of the spine, makes kneading motions using the first two fingers and thumb of each hand. Circles hands up along spine, circling at shoulders and buttocks.		
10.	Gently massages bony areas. Massages around any red areas, rather than on them.		
11.	Lets resident know when back rub is almost completed. Finishes with long smooth strokes.		
12.	Dries the back.		
13.	Removes blanket and towel, assists resident with getting dressed, and positions resident comfortably.		

14.	Stores lotion and disposes of dirty linens and clothing properly.		
15.	Returns bed to lowest position.		
16.	Places call light within resident's reach.		
17.	Washes hands.		
18.	Documents procedure.		

_____   _____
Date Reviewed   Instructor Signature

_____   _____
Date Performed   Instructor Signature

Shampooing hair

	Procedure Steps	yes	no
1.	Washes hands.		
2.	Identifies self by name. Identifies resident by name.		
3.	Explains procedure to resident, speaking clearly, slowly, and directly. Maintains face-to-face contact whenever possible.		
4.	Provides privacy.		
5.	Checks water temperature (105°F). Has resident test water temperature and adjusts if necessary.		
6.	Positions resident at sink or in bed, and wets hair.		
7.	Applies shampoo, and massages scalp.		
8.	Rinses hair thoroughly. Repeats. Uses conditioner if requested.		
9.	Wraps resident's hair.		
10.	Removes towel and combs/brushes hair.		
11.	Dries and styles hair.		
12.	Returns bed to lowest position if adjusted.		
13.	Places call light within resident's reach.		

14.	Washes and stores equipment.		
15.	Washes hands.		
16.	Documents procedure.		

_____   _____
Date Reviewed   Instructor Signature

_____   _____
Date Performed   Instructor Signature

Giving a shower or tub bath

	Procedure Steps	yes	no
1.	Washes hands. Places equipment in area. Cleans shower or tub area.		
2.	Washes hands.		
3.	Goes to resident's room. Identifies self by name. Identifies resident by name.		
4.	Explains procedure to resident. Speaks clearly, slowly, and directly. Maintains face-to-face contact whenever possible.		
5.	Provides privacy.		
6.	Helps resident put on nonskid footwear and transports to shower or tub room.		
	For a shower:		
7.	Places shower chair in position. Locks wheels. Transfers resident into chair.		
8.	Turns on water. Tests water temperature to make sure it is no more than 105°F. Has resident check water temperature.		
	For a tub bath:		
7.	Transfers resident onto chair or tub lift.		
8.	Fills tub halfway with warm water (105°F). Has resident check water temperature.		

Name: _____

	For either procedure:		
9.	Puts on gloves.		
10.	Helps resident remove clothing and shoes and get into shower or tub. Puts shower chair into shower and locks wheels.		
11.	Stays with resident during procedure. Lets resident wash as much as possible. Helps to wash his or her face. Helps to shampoo and rinse hair.		
12.	Helps to wash and rinse entire body, moving from head to toe.		
13.	Turns off water or drains tub. Covers resident with blanket.		
14.	Helps resident out of shower or tub and onto a chair. Gives resident a towel and helps to pat dry all areas of body.		
15.	Applies lotion and deodorant as needed.		
16.	Places soiled clothing and linen in proper containers.		
17.	Removes and disposes of gloves.		
18.	Washes hands.		
19.	Helps resident dress, comb hair, and put on footwear. Returns resident to his or her room.		
20.	Places call light within resident's reach.		
21.	Documents procedure.		

_____   _____
Date Reviewed   Instructor Signature

_____   _____
Date Performed   Instructor Signature

Providing fingernail care			
	Procedure Steps	yes	no
1.	Washes hands.		
2.	Identifies self by name. Identifies resident by name.		

3.	Explains procedure to resident, speaking clearly, slowly, and directly. Maintains face-to-face contact whenever possible.		
4.	Provides privacy.		
5.	Adjusts the bed to a safe working level, usually waist high. Locks bed wheels.		
6.	Fills basin halfway with warm water (105°F). Has resident test water temperature and adjusts if necessary.		
7.	Soaks all 10 fingertips for at least five minutes.		
8.	Removes hands from water. Washes hands with soapy washcloth. Rinses. Dries resident's hands with a towel, including between fingers.		
9.	Puts on gloves.		
10.	Uses pointed end of orangewood stick to remove dirt from under the nails. Wipes orangewood stick on towel after each nail. Washes the hands again and dries.		
11.	Shapes fingernails in a curve with an emery board or nail file. Finishes with nails free of rough edges. Applies lotion.		
12.	Discards water and rinses basin. Places basin in designated area and places soiled clothing and linens in proper containers.		
13.	Discards gloves and washes hands.		
14.	Returns bed to lowest position.		
15.	Places call light within resident's reach.		
16.	Washes hands.		
17.	Documents procedure.		

_____   _____
Date Reviewed   Instructor Signature

_____   _____
Date Performed   Instructor Signature

Providing foot care

	Procedure Steps	yes	no
1.	Washes hands.		
2.	Identifies self by name. Identifies resident by name.		
3.	Explains procedure to resident, speaking clearly, slowly, and directly. Maintains face-to-face contact whenever possible.		
4.	Provides privacy.		
5.	Adjusts the bed to a safe working level, usually waist high. Locks bed wheels.		
6.	Fills basin with warm water (105°F). Has resident test water temperature and adjusts if necessary.		
7.	Soaks resident's feet for five to ten minutes, adding warm water as necessary.		
8.	Puts on gloves.		
9.	Removes one foot from water. Washes entire foot, including between the toes and around nail beds with soapy washcloth.		
10.	Rinses and dries entire foot, including between the toes.		
11.	Repeats steps for other foot.		
12.	Applies lotion except for between the toes.		
13.	Discards water and rinses basin. Places basin in designated area and places soiled clothing and linens in proper containers.		
14.	Discards gloves and washes hands.		
15.	Returns bed to lowest position.		
16.	Places call light within resident's reach.		
17.	Washes hands.		

18.	Documents procedure.		

_____   _____
Date Reviewed   Instructor Signature

_____   _____
Date Performed   Instructor Signature

Shaving a resident

	Procedure Steps	yes	no
1.	Washes hands.		
2.	Identifies self by name. Identifies resident by name.		
3.	Explains procedure to resident, speaking clearly, slowly, and directly. Maintains face-to-face contact whenever possible.		
4.	Provides privacy.		
5.	Places equipment within reach. Adjusts bed to a safe working level, usually waist high. Raises head of bed so that resident is sitting up. Locks bed wheels.		
6.	Places towel across resident's chest, under the chin.		
7.	Puts on gloves.		
	If using a safety or disposable razor:		
8.	Softens beard and lathers face. Shaves in direction of hair growth, using downward strokes on face and upward strokes on neck. Rinses blade often. Rinses and dries face. Offers mirror.		
	If using an electric razor:		
8.	Cleans razor. Turns on, pulls skin taut, and shaves with smooth, even movements. Shaves beard with back and forth motion in direction of beard growth with foil shaver. Shaves beard in circular motion with three-head shaver. Shaves the chin and under the chin. Offers mirror.		

	Final steps:		
9.	Applies aftershave if resident desires.		
10.	Puts towel and linens in proper container. Cleans and stores equipment.		
11.	Removes and discards gloves. Washes hands.		
12.	Returns bed to lowest position.		
13.	Places call light within resident's reach.		
14.	Documents procedure.		

Date Reviewed _____ Instructor Signature _____

Date Performed _____ Instructor Signature _____

Combing or brushing hair

	Procedure Steps	yes	no
1.	Washes hands.		
2.	Identifies self by name. Identifies resident by name.		
3.	Explains procedure to resident, speaking clearly, slowly, and directly. Maintains face-to-face contact whenever possible.		
4.	Provides privacy.		
5.	Adjusts the bed to a safe working level, usually waist high. Locks bed wheels.		
6.	Raises head of bed so that resident is sitting up. Places towel under head or around shoulders. Removes hairpins, hair ties, and clips.		
7.	If hair is tangled, detangles gently.		
8.	Brushes hair from roots to ends in two-inch sections at a time.		
9.	Styles hair in the way the resident prefers. Offers a mirror to resident.		
10.	Returns bed to lowest position.		

11.	Places call light within resident's reach.		
12.	Returns supplies to storage and disposes of soiled linen in proper containers.		
13.	Washes hands.		
14.	Documents procedure.		

Date Reviewed _____ Instructor Signature _____

Date Performed _____ Instructor Signature _____

Dressing a resident with an affected (weak) right arm

	Procedure Steps	yes	no
	When putting on all items, moves resident's body gently and naturally. Avoids force and over-extension of limbs and joints.		
1.	Washes hands.		
2.	Identifies self by name. Identifies resident by name.		
3.	Explains procedure to resident. Speaks clearly, slowly, and directly. Maintains face-to-face contact whenever possible.		
4.	Provides privacy.		
5.	Asks resident which outfit she would like to wear. Dresses her in outfit of choice.		
6.	Removes resident's gown without completely exposing resident. Takes gown off stronger side first when undressing. Then removes gown from weaker side.		
7.	Helps resident to put the right (affected/weaker) arm through the right sleeve of the shirt, sweater, or slip before placing garment on left (unaffected) arm.		
8.	Assists resident to put on skirt, pants, or dress.		

9.	Places bed at lowest position. Locks bed wheels.		
10.	Applies non-skid footwear. Ties laces.		
11.	Finishes with resident dressed appropriately. Makes sure clothing is right-side-out and zippers/buttons are fastened.		
12.	Places gown in proper container.		
13.	Places call light within resident's reach.		
14.	Washes hands.		
15.	Reports any changes in resident.		
16.	Documents procedure.		

_____ _____
Date Reviewed   Instructor Signature

_____ _____
Date Performed   Instructor Signature

Providing oral care

	Procedure Steps	yes	no
1.	Washes hands.		
2.	Identifies self by name. Identifies resident by name.		
3.	Explains procedure to resident. Speaks clearly, slowly, and directly. Maintains face-to-face contact whenever possible.		
4.	Provides privacy.		
5.	Adjusts bed to a safe level, usually waist high. Locks bed wheels. Makes sure resident is in an upright sitting position.		
6.	Puts on gloves.		
7.	Places towel across resident's chest.		
8.	Wets brush and puts on small amount of toothpaste.		
9.	Cleans entire mouth (including tongue and all surfaces of teeth), using gentle strokes. First brushes upper teeth, then lower teeth.		

10.	Holds emesis basin to resident's chin. Has resident rinse mouth with water and spit into emesis basin. Wipes resident's mouth and removes towel.		
11.	Disposes of soiled linen in proper container.		
12.	Cleans and returns supplies to proper storage.		
13.	Removes and disposes of gloves. Washes hands.		
14.	Returns bed to lowest position.		
15.	Places call light within resident's reach.		
16.	Washes hands.		
17.	Documents procedure.		

_____ _____
Date Reviewed   Instructor Signature

_____ _____
Date Performed   Instructor Signature

Providing oral care for the unconscious resident

	Procedure Steps	yes	no
1.	Washes hands.		
2.	Identifies self by name. Identifies resident by name.		
3.	Explains procedure to resident. Speaks clearly, slowly, and directly. Maintains face-to-face contact whenever possible.		
4.	Provides for privacy.		
5.	Adjusts bed to a safe working level, usually waist high. Locks bed wheels.		
6.	Puts on gloves.		
7.	Turns resident's head to the side and places a towel under his cheek and chin. Places an emesis basin next to the cheek and chin.		
8.	Holds mouth open with padded tongue blade.		

Name: _____

		yes	no
9.	Dips swab in cleaning solution. Wipes teeth, gums, tongue, and inside surfaces of mouth, changing swab frequently. Repeats until the mouth is clean.		
10.	Rinses with clean swab dipped in water.		
11.	Removes the towel and basin. Pats lips or face dry if needed. Applies lip moisturizer.		
12.	Disposes of soiled linen in proper container. Cleans and returns supplies to proper storage.		
13.	Removes and disposes of gloves. Washes hands.		
14.	Returns bed to lowest position.		
15.	Places call light within resident's reach.		
16.	Washes hands.		
17.	Documents procedure.		

_____   _____
Date Reviewed   Instructor Signature

_____   _____
Date Performed   Instructor Signature

Flossing teeth

	Procedure Steps	yes	no
1.	Washes hands.		
2.	Identifies self by name. Identifies resident by name.		
3.	Explains procedure to resident. Speaks clearly, slowly, and directly. Maintains face-to-face contact whenever possible.		
4.	Provides for privacy.		
5.	Adjusts bed to a safe level, usually waist high. Locks bed wheels. Makes sure resident is in an upright sitting position.		
6.	Puts on gloves.		
7.	Wraps floss around index fingers.		

		yes	no
8.	Flosses teeth, starting with back and moving to gum line.		
9.	Uses clean area of floss after every two teeth.		
10.	Offers water periodically and offers a towel when done.		
11.	Discards floss, and cleans and stores supplies. Disposes of soiled linen in proper container.		
12.	Removes and disposes of gloves properly. Washes hands.		
13.	Returns bed to lowest position.		
14.	Places call light within resident's reach.		
15.	Washes hands.		
16.	Documents procedure.		

_____   _____
Date Reviewed   Instructor Signature

_____   _____
Date Performed   Instructor Signature

Cleaning and storing dentures

	Procedure Steps	yes	no
1.	Washes hands.		
2.	Puts on gloves.		
3.	Lines sink/basin with towels and fills with water.		
4.	Rinses dentures in cool running water before brushing them.		
5.	Applies toothpaste or cleanser to toothbrush.		
6.	Brushes dentures on all surfaces.		
7.	Rinses all surfaces of dentures under cool running water.		
8.	Rinses denture cup before placing clean dentures in it.		
9.	Places dentures in clean denture cup with solution or cool water. Makes sure cup is labeled with resident's name and room number.		

10.	Cleans and returns the equipment to proper storage.		
11.	Drains sink and disposes of towels in appropriate container.		
12.	Removes and disposes of gloves.		
13.	Washes hands.		
14.	Documents procedure.		

_____	_____
Date Reviewed	Instructor Signature
_____	_____
Date Performed	Instructor Signature

14
Basic Nursing Skills

Taking and recording an oral temperature			
	Procedure Steps	yes	no
1.	Washes hands.		
2.	Identifies self by name. Identifies resident by name.		
3.	Explains procedure to resident, speaking clearly, slowly, and directly. Maintains face-to-face contact whenever possible.		
4.	Provides privacy.		
5.	Puts on gloves.		
	Mercury-free thermometer:		
6.	Holds thermometer by stem. Shakes thermometer down to below the lowest number.		
	Digital thermometer:		
	Puts on disposable sheath. Turns on thermometer and waits until "ready" sign appears.		
	Electronic thermometer:		
	Removes probe from base unit and puts on probe cover.		
	Mercury-free thermometer:		
7.	Puts on disposable sheath, if available. Inserts bulb end of thermometer into resident's mouth, under tongue and to one side.		
	Digital thermometer:		
	Inserts end of digital thermometer into resident's mouth, under tongue and to one side.		
	Electronic thermometer:		
	Inserts end of electronic thermometer into resident's mouth, under tongue and to one side.		
	Mercury-free thermometer:		
8.	Instructs resident on how to hold thermometer in mouth. Leaves thermometer in place for at least three minutes.		
	Digital thermometer:		
	Leaves in place until thermometer blinks or beeps.		
	Electronic thermometer:		
	Leaves in place until tone or light signals temperature has been read.		
	Mercury-free thermometer:		
9.	Removes thermometer. Wipes with tissue from stem to bulb or removes sheath. Disposes of tissue or sheath. Reads temperature and remembers reading.		
	Digital thermometer:		
	Removes thermometer. Reads temperature on display screen and remembers reading.		
	Electronic thermometer:		
	Reads temperature on display screen and remembers reading.		
	Mercury-free thermometer:		
10.	Rinses and dries thermometer and stores properly.		

Name: _____

	Digital thermometer:		
	Removes and disposes of sheath with a tissue. Stores thermometer.		
	Electronic thermometer:		
	Presses the eject button to discard the cover. Returns probe to holder.		
11.	Removes and discards gloves.		
12	Washes hands.		
13.	Documents temperature, date, time, and method used.		
14.	Places call light within resident's reach.		

_____   _____
Date Reviewed   Instructor Signature

_____   _____
Date Performed   Instructor Signature

Taking and recording a rectal temperature			
	Procedure Steps	yes	no
1.	Washes hands.		
2.	Identifies self by name. Identifies resident by name.		
3.	Explains procedure to resident, speaking clearly, slowly, and directly. Maintains face-to-face contact whenever possible.		
4.	Provides privacy.		
5.	Adjusts bed to safe level, usually waist high. Locks bed wheels.		
6.	Assists resident to left-lying position.		
7.	Folds back linens to expose only rectal area.		
8.	Puts on gloves.		
	Mercury-free thermometer:		
9.	Holds thermometer by stem. Shakes thermometer down to below the lowest number.		

	Digital thermometer:		
	Puts on disposable sheath. Turns on thermometer and waits until "ready" sign appears.		
10.	Applies a small amount of lubricant to tip or bulb or probe cover.		
11.	Separates buttocks. Gently inserts thermometer into rectum one inch. Replaces sheet over buttocks. Holds onto thermometer at all times while taking temperature.		
	Mercury-free thermometer:		
12.	Holds thermometer in place for at least three minutes.		
	Digital thermometer:		
	Holds thermometer in place until thermometer blinks or beeps.		
13.	Removes thermometer and wipes thermometer with tissue from stem to bulb or removes sheath. Disposes of tissue or sheath.		
14.	Reads temperature and remembers reading.		
	Mercury-free thermometer:		
15.	Rinses and dries thermometer and stores properly.		
	Digital thermometer:		
	Discards probe cover and stores thermometer.		
16.	Removes and discards gloves.		
17.	Washes hands.		
18.	Documents temperature, date, time, and method used.		
19.	Places call light within resident's reach.		

_____   _____
Date Reviewed   Instructor Signature

_____   _____
Date Performed   Instructor Signature

Taking and recording a tympanic temperature

	Procedure Steps	yes	no
1.	Washes hands.		
2.	Identifies self by name. Identifies resident by name.		
3.	Explains procedure to resident, speaking clearly, slowly, and directly. Maintains face-to-face contact whenever possible.		
4.	Provides privacy.		
5.	Puts on gloves.		
6.	Places disposable sheath over earpiece of thermometer.		
7.	Positions resident's head properly and pulls up and back on the outside edge of the ear. Inserts covered probe and presses the button.		
8.	Holds thermometer in place for one second or until it beeps.		
9.	Reads temperature and remembers reading.		
10.	Discards sheath and stores thermometer properly.		
11.	Removes and discards gloves.		
12.	Washes hands.		
13.	Documents temperature, date, time, and method used.		
14.	Places call light within resident's reach.		

_____   _____
Date Reviewed   Instructor Signature

_____   _____
Date Performed   Instructor Signature

Taking and recording an axillary temperature

	Procedure Steps	yes	no
1.	Washes hands.		
2.	Identifies self by name. Identifies resident by name.		
3.	Explains procedure to resident, speaking clearly, slowly, and directly. Maintains face-to-face contact whenever possible.		
4.	Provides privacy.		
5.	Puts on gloves.		
6.	Removes resident's arm from sleeve and wipes axillary area with tissues.		
	Mercury-free thermometer:		
7.	Holds thermometer by stem. Shakes thermometer down to below the lowest number.		
	Digital thermometer:		
	Puts on disposable sheath. Turns on thermometer and waits until "ready" sign appears.		
	Electronic thermometer:		
	Removes probe from base unit and puts on probe cover.		
8.	Positions thermometer in center of armpit and folds resident's arm over chest.		
	Mercury-free thermometer:		
9.	Holds thermometer in place for eight to ten minutes.		
	Digital thermometer:		
	Leaves in place until thermometer blinks or beeps.		
	Electronic thermometer:		
	Leaves in place until tone or light signals temperature has been read.		
	Mercury-free thermometer:		
10.	Removes thermometer. Wipes with tissue from stem to bulb or removes sheath. Disposes of tissue or sheath. Reads temperature and remembers reading.		
	Digital thermometer:		
	Removes thermometer. Reads temperature on display screen and remembers reading.		

	Electronic thermometer:		
	Reads temperature on display screen and remembers reading.		
	Mercury-free thermometer:		
11.	Rinses and dries thermometer and stores properly.		
	Digital thermometer:		
	Removes and disposes of sheath with a tissue. Stores thermometer.		
	Electronic thermometer:		
	Presses the eject button to discard the cover. Returns probe to holder.		
12.	Removes and discards gloves.		
13.	Washes hands.		
14.	Puts resident's arm back into sleeve.		
15.	Documents temperature, date, time, and method used.		
16.	Places call light within resident's reach.		

_____   _____
Date Reviewed   Instructor Signature

_____   _____
Date Performed   Instructor Signature

6.	Counts heartbeats for one minute.		
7.	Counts resident's respirations with stethoscope still in place.		
8.	Documents pulse rate, date, time, and method used. Notes any irregularities in rhythm.		
9.	Cleans earpieces and diaphragm of stethoscope. Stores stethoscope.		
10.	Washes hands.		
11.	Places call light within resident's reach.		

_____   _____
Date Reviewed   Instructor Signature

_____   _____
Date Performed   Instructor Signature

Taking and recording apical pulse

	Procedure Steps	yes	no
1.	Washes hands.		
2.	Identifies self by name. Identifies resident by name.		
3.	Explains procedure to resident, speaking clearly, slowly, and directly. Maintains face-to-face contact whenever possible.		
4.	Provides privacy.		
5.	Fits earpieces of stethoscope snugly in ears and places metal diaphragm on left side of chest, just below the nipple.		

Taking and recording radial pulse and counting and recording respirations

	Procedure Steps	yes	no
1.	Washes hands.		
2.	Identifies self by name. Identifies resident by name.		
3.	Explains procedure to resident, speaking clearly, slowly, and directly. Maintains face-to-face contact whenever possible.		
4.	Provides privacy.		
5.	Places fingertips on the thumb side of resident's wrist to locate pulse.		
6.	Counts beats for one full minute.		
7.	Keeping fingertips on resident's wrist, counts respirations for one full minute.		
8.	Documents pulse rate, date, time, and method used. Documents respiratory rate and the pattern or character of breathing.		

		yes	no
9.	Places call light within resident's reach.		
10.	Washes hands.		

_____   _____
Date Reviewed   Instructor Signature

_____   _____
Date Performed   Instructor Signature

Taking and recording blood pressure (one-step method)

	Procedure Steps	yes	no
1.	Washes hands.		
2.	Identifies self by name. Identifies resident by name.		
3.	Explains procedure to resident, speaking clearly, slowly, and directly. Maintains face-to-face contact whenever possible.		
4.	Provides privacy.		
5.	Asks resident to roll up sleeve. Positions resident's arm with palm up. The arm should be level with the heart.		
6.	With the valve open, squeezes the cuff to make sure it is completely deflated.		
7.	Places blood pressure cuff snugly on resident's upper arm, with the center of the cuff placed over the brachial artery.		
8.	Wipes diaphragm and earpieces of stethoscope with alcohol wipes.		
9.	Locates the brachial pulse with fingertips. Places diaphragm of stethoscope over brachial artery, and places earpieces of stethoscope in ears.		
10.	Closes the valve (clockwise) until it stops. Does not tighten it.		
11.	Inflates cuff to 30 mmHg above the point at which the pulse is last heard or felt.		

12.	Opens the valve slightly with thumb and index finger. Deflates cuff slowly.		
13.	Watches gauge and listens for sound of pulse.		
14.	Remembers the reading at which the first clear pulse sound is heard. This is the systolic pressure.		
15.	Continues listening for a change or muffling of pulse sound. The point of a change or the point the sound disappears is the diastolic pressure. Remembers this reading.		
16.	Opens the valve to deflate cuff completely. Removes cuff.		
17.	Documents both systolic and diastolic pressures. Notes which arm was used.		
18.	Cleans stethoscope. Stores equipment.		
19.	Places call light within resident's reach.		
20.	Washes hands.		

_____   _____
Date Reviewed   Instructor Signature

_____   _____
Date Performed   Instructor Signature

Taking and recording blood pressure (two-step method)

	Procedure Steps	yes	no
1.	Washes hands.		
2.	Identifies self by name. Identifies resident by name.		
3.	Explains procedure to resident, speaking clearly, slowly, and directly. Maintains face-to-face contact whenever possible.		
4.	Provides privacy.		

Name: _____

5.	Asks resident to roll up sleeve. Positions resident's arm with palm up. The arm should be level with the heart.		
6.	With the valve open, squeezes the cuff to make sure it is completely deflated.		
7.	Places blood pressure cuff snugly on resident's upper arm, with the center of the cuff placed over the brachial artery.		
8.	Locates the radial (wrist) pulse with fingertips.		
9.	Closes the valve (clockwise) until it stops. Inflates cuff, watching gauge.		
10.	Stops inflating cuff when pulse is no longer felt. Notes the reading.		
11.	Opens the valve to deflate cuff completely. Removes cuff.		
12.	Writes down the estimated systolic reading.		
13.	Wipes diaphragm and earpieces of stethoscope with alcohol wipes.		
14.	Locates brachial pulse with fingertips.		
15.	Places earpieces of stethoscope in ears and places diaphragm of stethoscope over brachial artery.		
16.	Closes the valve (clockwise) until it stops. Does not tighten it.		
17.	Inflates cuff to 30 mmHg above the estimated systolic pressure.		
18.	Opens the valve slightly with thumb and index finger. Deflates cuff slowly.		
19.	Watches gauge and listens for sound of pulse.		
20.	Remembers the reading at which the first clear pulse sound is heard. This is the systolic pressure.		

21.	Continues listening for a change or muffling of pulse sound. The point of a change or the point the sound disappears is the diastolic pressure. Remembers this reading.		
22.	Opens the valve to deflate cuff completely. Removes cuff.		
23.	Documents both systolic and diastolic pressures. Notes which arm was used.		
24.	Cleans stethoscope. Stores equipment.		
25.	Places call light within resident's reach.		
26.	Washes hands.		

_____   _____
Date Reviewed   Instructor Signature

_____   _____
Date Performed   Instructor Signature

Applying warm compresses

	Procedure Steps	yes	no
1.	Washes hands.		
2.	Identifies self by name. Identifies resident by name.		
3.	Explains procedure to resident, speaking clearly, slowly, and directly. Maintains face-to-face contact whenever possible.		
4.	Provides privacy.		
5.	Fills basin one-half to two-thirds with hot water (105°F). Has resident check water temperature and adjusts if necessary.		
6.	Soaks wash cloth, wrings it out, and applies to area needing compress. Covers with plastic wrap and towel.		
7.	Notes the time. Checks area every five minutes. Removes compress if redness, numbness, pain, or discomfort occur. Changes compress if cooling occurs.		

8.	Removes compress after 20 minutes.		
9.	Discards water. Cleans and stores basin and other supplies properly. Places soiled towels in proper container, and discards plastic wrap.		
10.	Places call light within resident's reach.		
11.	Washes hands.		
12.	Documents procedure.		

_____   _____
Date Reviewed   Instructor Signature

_____   _____
Date Performed   Instructor Signature

10.	Removes basin and dries the resident with towel.		
11.	Discards water. Cleans and stores basin and other supplies properly. Places soiled towels in proper container.		
12.	Places call light within resident's reach.		
13.	Washes hands.		
14.	Documents procedure.		

_____   _____
Date Reviewed   Instructor Signature

_____   _____
Date Performed   Instructor Signature

Administering warm soaks

	Procedure Steps	yes	no
1.	Washes hands.		
2.	Identifies self by name. Identifies resident by name.		
3.	Explains procedure to resident, speaking clearly, slowly, and directly. Maintains face-to-face contact whenever possible.		
4.	Provides privacy.		
5.	Fills the basin half full of warm water (105°F). Has resident check water temperature and adjusts if necessary.		
6.	Immerses body part in water properly, padding the edge of the basin as necessary. Covers resident for extra warmth if needed.		
7.	Checks water temperature every five minutes, adding hot water as needed.		
8.	Observes area for redness and discontinues soak if resident complains of pain or discomfort.		
9.	Soaks for 15 to 20 minutes or as ordered in the care plan.		

Applying an Aquamatic K-Pad ®

	Procedure Steps	yes	no
1.	Washes hands.		
2.	Identifies self by name. Identifies resident by name.		
3.	Explains procedure to resident. Speaks clearly, slowly, and directly. Maintains face-to-face contact whenever possible.		
4.	Provides for privacy.		
5.	Adjusts bed to a safe level. Locks bed wheels.		
6.	Places unit on bedside table. Checks to make sure cords are not damaged and that tubing is intact.		
7.	Removes cover of control unit. Fills with distilled water to fill line if water level is low.		
8.	Puts cover of unit back on. Plugs unit in and turns pad on.		
9.	Places pad in cover.		
10.	Uncovers area to be treated. Places the pad and notes the time.		
11.	Returns to check area every five minutes, removing the pad if area is red or numb or if resident reports pain or discomfort.		

	Procedure Steps		
12.	Fills with distilled water when necessary.		
13.	Removes pad after 20 minutes.		
14.	Cleans and stores supplies.		
15.	Returns bed to lowest position.		
16.	Places call light within resident's reach.		
17.	Washes hands.		
18.	Documents procedure.		

_____   _____
Date Reviewed   Instructor Signature

_____   _____
Date Performed   Instructor Signature

Assisting with a sitz bath

	Procedure Steps	yes	no
1.	Washes hands.		
2.	Identifies self by name. Identifies resident by name.		
3.	Explains procedure to resident, speaking clearly, slowly, and directly. Maintains face-to-face contact whenever possible.		
4.	Provides privacy.		
5.	Puts on gloves.		
6.	Fills sitz bath two-thirds full with hot water (105°F).		
7.	Places sitz bath on toilet seat and helps resident undress and sit down on sitz bath.		
8.	Leaves the room and checks on resident every five minutes for weakness or dizziness. Stays with resident who is unsteady.		
9.	Assists resident out of sitz bath after 20 minutes. Provides towels and helps with dressing as needed.		
10.	Cleans and stores supplies.		
11.	Removes and discards gloves.		
12.	Washes hands.		

	Procedure Steps		
13.	Places call light within resident's reach.		
14.	Documents procedure.		

_____   _____
Date Reviewed   Instructor Signature

_____   _____
Date Performed   Instructor Signature

Applying ice packs

	Procedure Steps	yes	no
1.	Washes hands.		
2.	Identifies self by name. Identifies resident by name.		
3.	Explains procedure to resident, speaking clearly, slowly, and directly. Maintains face-to-face contact whenever possible.		
4.	Provides privacy.		
5.	Fills plastic bag or ice pack one-half to two-thirds full with ice and removes excess air. Covers bag with towel.		
6.	Applies bag to the area as ordered. Uses another towel to cover bag if it is too cold.		
7.	Notes the time and checks the area after 10 minutes for blisters or pale, white, or gray skin. Stops treatment if resident complains of numbness or pain.		
8.	Removes ice after 20 minutes or as ordered.		
9.	Stores ice pack and places towel in proper container.		
10.	Places call light within resident's reach.		
11.	Washes hands.		
12.	Documents procedure.		

_____   _____
Date Reviewed   Instructor Signature

_____   _____
Date Performed   Instructor Signature

Applying cold compresses

	Procedure Steps	yes	no
1.	Washes hands.		
2.	Identifies self by name. Identifies resident by name.		
3.	Explains procedure to resident, speaking clearly, slowly, and directly. Maintains face-to-face contact whenever possible.		
4.	Provides privacy.		
5.	Places bed protector. Rinses washcloth in basin, and wrings out washcloth.		
6.	Covers the area with sheet or towel and applies cold wash-cloth to the area. Changes wash-cloths to keep area cold.		
7.	Checks the area after five min-utes for blisters or pale, white, or gray skin. Stops treatment if resident complains of numb-ness or pain.		
8.	Removes compresses after 20 minutes or as ordered. Gives resident towels as needed to dry the area.		
9.	Cleans and stores basin prop-erly. Places towels in proper container.		
10.	Places call light within resident's reach.		
11.	Washes hands.		
12.	Documents procedure.		

_____   _____
Date Reviewed   Instructor Signature

_____   _____
Date Performed   Instructor Signature

Changing a dry dressing using non-sterile technique

	Procedure Steps	yes	no
1.	Washes hands.		
2.	Identifies self by name. Identifies resident by name.		
3.	Explains procedure to resident, speaking clearly, slowly, and directly. Maintains face-to-face contact whenever possible.		
4.	Provides privacy.		
5.	Cuts pieces of tape long enough to secure the dressing. Opens gauze package without touching the gauze. Places open package on flat surface.		
6.	Puts on gloves.		
7.	Removes soiled dressing gently by peeling tape toward wound. Lifts dressing off the wound and observes dressing for odor or drainage. Notes color and size of the wound. Disposes of used dressing in proper container. Removes and discards gloves.		
8.	Puts on new gloves.		
9.	Applies clean gauze to wound. Tapes gauze in place.		
10.	Removes and disposes of gloves.		
11.	Washes hands.		
12.	Places call light within resident's reach.		
13.	Documents procedure.		

_____   _____
Date Reviewed   Instructor Signature

_____   _____
Date Performed   Instructor Signature

Assisting in changing clothes for a resident who has an IV

	Procedure Steps	yes	no
1.	Washes hands.		
2.	Identifies self by name. Identifies resident by name.		

3.	Explains procedure to resident, speaking clearly, slowly, and directly. Maintains face-to-face contact whenever possible.		
4.	Provides privacy.		
5.	Adjusts bed to lowest position and locks bed wheels. Helps resident to sitting position with feet flat on the floor.		
6.	Helps resident remove the arm without the IV from the clothing.		
7.	Helps resident gather clothing on arm with IV site, lift clothing over IV site, and move it up the tubing toward the IV bag.		
8.	Lifts IV bag off the pole, keeping it higher than the IV site, slides clothing over IV bag, and replaces IV bag on the pole.		
9.	Sets used clothing aside and gathers the sleeve of the clean clothing.		
10.	Lifts IV bag off the pole again, keeping it higher than the IV site, slides clean clothing over IV bag onto the resident's arm, and replaces IV bag on the pole.		
11.	Moves clean clothing over tubing and IV site and onto the resident's arm.		
12.	Assists resident with putting other arm into clothing.		
13.	Checks the IV, the tubing, and dressing for proper placement.		
14.	Assists resident with changing the rest of the clothing.		
15.	Places soiled clothes in proper container.		
16.	Places call light within resident's reach.		
17.	Washes hands.		
18.	Documents procedure.		

_____ _____
Date Reviewed   Instructor Signature

_____ _____
Date Performed   Instructor Signature

15
Nutrition and Hydration

Feeding a resident who cannot feed self		
Procedure Steps	yes	no
1. Washes hands.		
2. Identifies self by name. Identifies resident by name.		
3. Explains procedure to resident. Speaks clearly, slowly, and directly. Maintains face-to-face contact whenever possible.		
4. Picks up diet card and asks resident to state his name. Verifies that resident has received the right tray.		
5. Raises the head of the bed. Makes sure resident is in an upright sitting position.		
6. Adjusts bed height to seat self at resident's eye level. Locks bed wheels.		
7. Helps resident wash hands if needed.		
8. Places meal tray where it can be easily seen by resident, such as on overbed table.		
9. Helps resident to put on clothing protector, if desired.		
10. Sits facing resident, at resident's eye level, on resident's stronger side.		
11. Tells resident what foods are on tray and asks what resident would like to eat first.		
12. Offers the food in bite-sized pieces, telling resident content of each bite offered. Alternates types of food offered, allowing for resident's preferences.		
13. Offers drink of beverage throughout the meal.		
14. Makes sure resident's mouth is empty before next bite of food or sip of beverage.		

		yes	no
15.	Talks with resident during meal.		
16.	Wipes food from resident's mouth and hands as necessary during the meal. Wipes again at the end of the meal.		
17.	Removes and disposes of clothing protector if used.		
18.	Removes food tray, checking for personal items. Places tray in proper area.		
19.	Returns bed to lowest position.		
20.	Places call light within resident's reach.		
21.	Washes hands.		
22.	Documents procedure.		

_____   _____
Date Reviewed   Instructor Signature

_____   _____
Date Performed   Instructor Signature

Measuring and recording intake and output

	Procedure Steps	yes	no
1.	Washes hands.		
2.	Identifies self by name. Identifies resident by name.		
3.	Explains procedure to resident, speaking clearly, slowly, and directly. Maintains face-to-face contact whenever possible.		
4.	Provides privacy.		
5.	Measures amount of fluid resident is served and notes on paper.		
6.	Measures leftover fluids and notes on paper.		
7.	Subtracts amount left over from amount served. Converts to milliliters.		
8.	Documents amount of fluids consumed (in mL) in input column in I&O sheet. Records time and what fluid was taken.		

		yes	no
9.	Washes hands.		
	For measuring the resident's output:		
1.	Washes hands.		
2.	Puts on gloves.		
3.	Pours contents of bedpan or urinal into measuring container.		
4.	Measures amount of urine, keeping container level.		
5.	Discards urine without splashing. Washes and stores equipment properly. Returns to proper storage.		
6.	Removes and discards gloves.		
7.	Washes hands.		
8.	Documents the time and amount (in mL) of urine in output column.		

_____   _____
Date Reviewed   Instructor Signature

_____   _____
Date Performed   Instructor Signature

Serving fresh water

	Procedure Steps	yes	no
1.	Washes hands.		
2.	Identifies self by name. Identifies resident by name.		
3.	Puts on gloves.		
4.	Scoops ice into water pitcher. Adds fresh water.		
5.	Uses and stores ice scoop properly.		
6.	Takes pitcher to resident. Pours glass of water for resident and leaves pitcher and glass at bedside.		
7.	Makes sure pitcher and glass are light enough for resident to lift. Leaves a straw if resident wants one.		
8.	Places call light within resident's reach.		

Name: _____

		yes	no
9.	Removes and discards gloves.		
10.	Washes hands.		

_____   _____
Date Reviewed   Instructor Signature

_____   _____
Date Performed   Instructor Signature

16
Urinary Elimination

Assisting a resident with the use of a bedpan

	Procedure Steps	yes	no
1.	Washes hands.		
2.	Identifies self by name. Identifies resident by name.		
3.	Explains procedure to resident, speaking clearly, slowly, and directly. Maintains face-to-face contact whenever possible.		
4.	Provides privacy.		
5.	Adjusts the bed to a safe working level, usually waist high. Locks bed wheels. Lowers head of bed.		
6.	Puts on gloves.		
7.	Covers resident with bath blanket. Places a protective pad under resident's buttocks and hips.		
8.	Asks resident to remove undergarments or assists resident to do so.		
9.	Places bedpan near hips in correct position (standard bedpan positioned with wider end aligned with the buttocks; fracture pan positioned with handle toward foot of bed). Slides bedpan under hips, helping resident if necessary.		
10.	Removes and discards gloves. Washes hands.		

		yes	no
11.	Raises head of bed and proper resident into semi-sitting position with pillows.		
12.	Checks bedpan position, ensuring blanket is covering resident. Provides resident with supplies and asks resident to clean hands with wipe when finished.		
13.	Places call light within reach and leaves room until resident calls.		
14.	When called, returns and puts on clean gloves. Lowers head of bed. Removes and covers bedpan.		
15.	If resident is unable, cleans the perineum properly. Assists with putting undergarments on. Places towel in bag and discards disposable supplies.		
16.	Takes bedpan to bathroom and empties bedpan into toilet. Rinses bedpan and empties rinse water into toilet. Places in proper area for cleaning.		
17.	Removes and discards gloves.		
18.	Washes hands.		
19.	Returns bed to lowest position.		
20.	Places call light within resident's reach.		
21.	Documents procedure.		

_____   _____
Date Reviewed   Instructor Signature

_____   _____
Date Performed   Instructor Signature

Assisting a male resident with a urinal

	Procedure Steps	yes	no
1.	Washes hands.		
2.	Identifies self by name. Identifies resident by name.		

	Procedure Steps	yes	no
3.	Explains procedure to resident, speaking clearly, slowly, and directly. Maintains face-to-face contact whenever possible.		
4.	Provides privacy.		
5.	Adjusts the bed to a safe working level, usually waist high. Locks bed wheels.		
6.	Puts on gloves.		
7.	Places protective pad under buttocks and hips.		
8.	Hands urinal to resident or places it if resident is unable. Replaces covers.		
9.	Removes and discards gloves. Washes hands.		
10.	Asks resident to clean hands with wipe when finished. Places call light within reach and leaves room until resident calls.		
11.	When called, returns and puts on clean gloves.		
12.	Removes urinal when resident is finished. Discards urine and rinses urinal. Places in proper area for cleaning.		
13.	Removes and discards gloves.		
14.	Washes hands.		
15.	Returns bed to lowest position.		
16.	Places call light within resident's reach.		
17.	Documents procedure.		

_____   _____
Date Reviewed   Instructor Signature

_____   _____
Date Performed   Instructor Signature

Assisting a resident to use a portable commode or toilet

	Procedure Steps	yes	no
1.	Washes hands.		

	Procedure Steps	yes	no
2.	Identifies self by name. Identifies resident by name.		
3.	Explains procedure to resident, speaking clearly, slowly, and directly. Maintains face-to-face contact whenever possible.		
4.	Provides privacy.		
5.	Helps resident to bathroom or commode.		
6.	Helps resident remove clothing and sit on toilet set. Puts toilet tissue within reach.		
7.	Leaves room or area, leaving call light within reach.		
8.	When called, returns and applies gloves.		
9.	Cleans perineal area if assistance is needed. Helps resident up and ensures resident's hands are washed.		
10.	Helps resident back to bed.		
11.	Removes waste container and empties into toilet. Rinses container and places container in proper area for cleaning.		
12.	Removes gloves and discards them.		
13.	Washes hands.		
14.	Returns bed to lowest position.		
15.	Places call light within resident's reach.		
16.	Documents procedure.		

_____   _____
Date Reviewed   Instructor Signature

_____   _____
Date Performed   Instructor Signature

Providing perineal care for an incontinent resident

	Procedure Steps	yes	no
1.	Washes hands.		
2.	Identifies self by name. Identifies resident by name.		

3.	Explains procedure to resident. Speaks clearly, slowly, and directly. Maintains face-to-face contact whenever possible.		
4.	Provides privacy.		
5.	Adjusts bed to a safe working level, usually waist high. Locks bed wheels. Lowers head of bed and positions resident lying flat on his back.		
6.	Tests water temperature with thermometer or wrist. Water temperature should be 105°F. Has resident check water temperature. Adjusts if necessary.		
7.	Puts on gloves.		
8.	Covers resident with bath blanket, and moves top linens to foot of bed.		
9.	Removes soiled protective pad from underneath resident by turning resident on his side, away from self. Rolls soiled pad into itself with wet side in/dry side out.		
10.	Places clean protective pad under buttocks.		
11.	Returns resident to lying on his back.		
12.	Exposes perineal area only. Cleans perineal area from front to back.		
13.	Turns resident on his side away from self. Removes the wet protective pad after drying buttocks.		
14.	Places a dry protective pad underneath resident. Repositions resident.		
15.	Replaces top covers, removes bath blanket, and places soiled clothing, linens, and protective pads in proper containers.		
16.	Empties, rinses, and wipes basin and returns to proper storage.		
17.	Removes and disposes of gloves properly.		

18.	Washes hands.		
19.	Returns bed to lowest position.		
20.	Places call light within resident's reach.		
21.	Documents procedure.		

_____ Date Reviewed _____ Instructor Signature

_____ Date Performed _____ Instructor Signature

Providing catheter care

	Procedure Steps	yes	no
1.	Washes hands.		
2.	Identifies self by name. Identifies resident by name.		
3.	Explains procedure to resident, speaking clearly, slowly, and directly. Maintains face-to-face contact whenever possible.		
4.	Provides privacy.		
5.	Adjusts the bed to safe working level, usually waist high. Locks bed wheels. Lowers head of bed and positions resident lying flat on back.		
6.	Removes or folds back top bedding, keeping resident covered with bath blanket.		
7.	Tests water temperature with thermometer or wrist. Water temperature should be 105°F. Has resident check water temperature. Adjusts if necessary.		
8.	Puts on gloves.		
9.	Places clean protective pad under buttocks.		
10.	Exposes only the area necessary to clean the catheter.		
11.	Places towel or pad under catheter tubing before washing.		
12.	Applies soap to washcloth and cleans area around meatus, using a clean area of the cloth for each stroke.		

13.	Holding catheter near meatus, cleans at least four inches of catheter. Moves in only one direction, away from meatus. Uses a clean area of the cloth for each stroke.		
14.	Rinses area around meatus and rinses at least four inches of catheter nearest meatus, moving away from meatus. Uses a clean area of the cloth for each stroke.		
15.	Removes towel or pad and bath blanket, and replaces top covers.		
16.	Disposes of linen in proper containers. Empties and rinses basin. Returns to storage.		
17.	Removes and discards gloves.		
18.	Washes hands.		
19.	Returns bed to lowest position.		
20.	Places call light within resident's reach.		
21.	Documents procedure.		

_____   _____
Date Reviewed   Instructor Signature

_____   _____
Date Performed   Instructor Signature

Emptying the catheter drainage bag

	Procedure Steps	yes	no
1.	Washes hands.		
2.	Identifies self by name. Identifies resident by name.		
3.	Explains procedure to resident. Speaks clearly, slowly, and directly. Maintains face-to-face contact whenever possible.		
4.	Provides privacy.		
5.	Puts on gloves.		
6.	Places measuring container on paper towel on floor.		

7.	Opens drain or spout on bag so urine flows into measuring container.		
8.	Closes spout and cleans it. Replaces drain in its holder on the bag.		
9.	Notes amount and appearance of urine and empties it into toilet.		
10.	Cleans and stores measuring container properly.		
11.	Removes and discards gloves.		
12.	Washes hands.		
13.	Documents procedure.		

_____   _____
Date Reviewed   Instructor Signature

_____   _____
Date Performed   Instructor Signature

Applying a condom catheter

	Procedure Steps	yes	no
1.	Washes hands.		
2.	Identifies self by name. Identifies resident by name.		
3.	Explains procedure to resident, speaking clearly, slowly, and directly. Maintains face-to-face contact whenever possible.		
4.	Provides privacy.		
5.	Adjusts the bed to a safe working level, usually waist high. Locks bed wheels. Lowers head of bed and positions resident lying flat on back.		
6.	Removes or folds back bedding, keeping resident covered with bath blanket.		
7.	Puts on gloves.		
8.	Adjusts bath blanket to expose only genital area.		

9.	Removes condom catheter if one is in place.		
10.	Assists as necessary with perineal care.		
11.	Attaches collection bag to leg.		
12.	Moves pubic hair away from penis. Places condom on penis and rolls toward base of penis, leaving space between drainage tip and glans of penis to prevent irritation.		
13.	Gently secures a condom to penis.		
14.	Connects catheter tip to drainage tubing. Makes sure tubing is not twisted or kinked.		
15.	Discards used supplies in plastic bag. Places soiled linen and clothing in proper containers.		
16.	Removes and discards gloves.		
17.	Washes hands.		
18.	Returns bed to its lowest position.		
19.	Places call light within resident's reach.		
20.	Documents procedure.		

_____ _____
Date Reviewed   Instructor Signature

_____ _____
Date Performed   Instructor Signature

6.	Assists resident to bathroom or commode, or offers bedpan or urinal.		
7.	Has resident void. Asks resident not to put toilet paper in with the sample. Provides a plastic bag to discard toilet paper separately.		
8.	Assists as necessary with perineal care. Helps resident wash his or her hands.		
9.	Takes bedpan, urinal, or commode pail to the bathroom.		
10.	Pours urine into specimen container, making it at least half full.		
11.	Covers container with lid. Wipes off the outside with a paper towel.		
12.	Places the container in a plastic bag.		
13.	Discards extra urine. Rinses and cleans equipment, and stores it.		
14.	Removes and discards gloves.		
15.	Washes hands.		
16.	Returns bed to lowest position.		
17.	Places call light within resident's reach.		
18.	Takes specimen and lab slip to proper area. Documents procedure.		

_____ _____
Date Reviewed   Instructor Signature

_____ _____
Date Performed   Instructor Signature

Collecting a routine urine specimen

	Procedure Steps	yes	no
1.	Washes hands.		
2.	Identifies self by name. Identifies resident by name.		
3.	Explains procedure to resident, speaking clearly, slowly, and directly. Maintains face-to-face contact whenever possible.		
4.	Provides privacy.		
5.	Puts on gloves.		

Collecting a clean catch (mid-stream) urine specimen

	Procedure Steps	yes	no
1.	Washes hands.		
2.	Identifies self by name. Identifies resident by name.		

3.	Explains procedure to resident, speaking clearly, slowly, and directly. Maintains face-to-face contact whenever possible.		
4.	Provides privacy.		
5.	Puts on gloves.		
6.	Opens specimen kit.		
7.	Cleans the area around the meatus or head of the penis.		
8.	Asks resident to urinate into the bedpan, urinal, or toilet, and to stop before urination is complete.		
9.	Places container under the urine stream and instructs resident to start urinating again until container is at least half full. Has resident finish urinating in bedpan, urinal, or toilet.		
10.	Covers urine container and wipes off outside with paper towel. Places in a plastic bag.		
11.	Discards extra urine. Rinses, cleans, and stores equipment.		
12.	Assists as necessary with perineal care.		
13.	Removes gloves.		
14.	Washes hands. Assists resident to wash hands.		
15.	Returns bed to lowest position.		
16.	Places call light within resident's reach.		
17.	Takes specimen and lab slip to proper area. Documents procedure.		

_____   _____
Date Reviewed   Instructor Signature

_____   _____
Date Performed   Instructor Signature

Collecting a 24-hour urine specimen

	Procedure Steps	yes	no
1.	Washes hands.		

2.	Identifies self by name. Identifies resident by name.		
3.	Explains procedure to resident. Speaks clearly, slowly, and directly. Maintains face-to-face contact whenever possible. Emphasizes that all urine must be saved.		
4.	Provides privacy.		
5.	Places sign on bed indicating all urine within 24 hours is being collected.		
6.	Instructs resident to completely empty the bladder. Discards urine and notes the exact time.		
7.	Labels container with resident's name, room number, and dates and times.		
8.	Puts on gloves each time resident voids.		
9.	Pours urine into container.		
10.	Helps with perineal care as needed. Helps resident to wash hands after each voiding.		
11.	Cleans equipment after each voiding.		
12.	Removes gloves.		
13.	Washes hands.		
14.	After last void, adds urine to container. Removes sign.		
15.	Places container in plastic bag. Removes and disposes of gloves.		
16.	Washes hands.		
17.	Makes resident comfortable.		
18.	Returns bed to lowest position.		
19.	Places call light within resident's reach.		
20.	Takes specimen and lab slip to proper area. Documents procedure.		

_____   _____
Date Reviewed   Instructor Signature

_____   _____
Date Performed   Instructor Signature

Testing urine with reagent strips

	Procedure Steps	yes	no
1.	Washes hands.		
2.	Puts on gloves.		
3.	Takes strip and recaps bottle, closing bottle tightly.		
4.	Dips strip into specimen.		
5.	Removes strip at correct time.		
6.	Compares strip with color chart on bottle.		
7.	Reads results.		
8.	Discards used items. Discards specimen in toilet.		
9.	Removes gloves.		
10.	Washes hands.		
11.	Documents procedure.		

_____   _____
Date Reviewed   Instructor Signature

_____   _____
Date Performed   Instructor Signature

17
Bowel Elimination

Giving a cleansing enema

	Procedure Steps	yes	no
1.	Washes hands.		
2.	Identifies self by name. Identifies resident by name.		
3.	Explains procedure to resident. Speaks clearly, slowly, and directly. Maintains face-to-face contact whenever possible.		
4.	Provides privacy.		
5.	Adjusts bed to a safe level, usually waist high. Locks bed wheels.		
6.	Raises side rail on far side of bed. Lowers side rail nearest self.		

7.	Helps resident into left-sided Sims' position. Covers with a bath blanket.		
8.	Places IV pole beside the bed. Raises side rail.		
9.	Clamps enema tube. Prepares enema solution. Fills bag with 500-1000 mL of warm water (105°F). Mixes solution.		
10.	Unclamps tube. Lets a small amount of solution run through tubing. Re-clamps tube.		
11.	Hangs bag on IV pole. Makes sure bottom of bag is not more than 12 inches above the resident's anus.		
12.	Puts on gloves.		
13.	Lowers side rail. Uncovers enough to expose anus only.		
14.	Places bed protector under resident. Places bedpan close to resident's body.		
15.	Lubricates tip of tubing. Asks resident to breathe deeply.		
16.	Lifts buttock to expose anus and asks resident to take a deep breath and exhale.		
17.	Gently inserts tip of tubing two to four inches into rectum.		
18.	Unclamps tubing. Allows solution to flow slowly. Encourages resident to take as much of solution as possible.		
19.	Clamps the tubing when solution is almost gone. Removes tip from rectum and places it into enema bag. Does not contaminate self, resident, or linens.		
20.	Asks the resident to hold solution inside as long as possible.		
21.	Helps resident to use bedpan, commode, or get to bathroom.		

22.	Places call light and toilet tissue or wipes within resident's reach. Asks resident to clean hands with wipes if able. Asks resident to signal when finished and leaves room.		
23.	Discards disposable equipment. Cleans area.		
24.	Removes gloves and washes hands.		
25.	When called, returns and puts on clean gloves. Helps with perineal care as needed.		
26.	Removes bedpan. Removes bed protector.		
27.	Empties bedpan if used. Checks bedpan or toilet for consistency, color, and amount of stool.		
28.	Rinses bedpan and places in proper area for cleaning.		
29.	Removes and discards gloves		
30.	Washes hands.		
31.	Removes bath blanket. Returns bed to proper position.		
32.	Places call light within resident's reach.		
33.	Documents procedure.		

_____   _____
Date Reviewed   Instructor Signature

_____   _____
Date Performed   Instructor Signature

Giving a commercial enema

	Procedure Steps	yes	no
1.	Washes hands.		
2.	Identifies self by name. Identifies resident by name.		
3.	Explains procedure to resident. Speaks clearly, slowly, and directly. Maintains face-to-face contact whenever possible.		
4.	Provides privacy.		

5.	Adjusts bed to a safe level, usually waist high. Locks bed wheels.		
6.	Raises side rail on far side of bed. Lowers side rail nearest self.		
7.	Helps resident into left-sided Sims' position. Covers with a bath blanket.		
8.	Puts on gloves.		
9.	Uncovers resident enough to expose anus only. Places bed protector under resident. Places bedpan close to resident's body.		
10.	Lubricates tip of bottle.		
11.	Asks resident to breathe deeply during procedure.		
12.	Lifts buttock to expose anus and asks resident to take a deep breath and exhale. Gently inserts tip of tubing one and a half inches into rectum.		
13.	Slowly squeezes and rolls container so that solution runs inside the resident.		
14.	Removes tip and places bottle inside box upside-down.		
15.	Asks resident to hold solution inside as long as possible.		
16.	Helps resident to use bedpan, commode, or get to bathroom.		
17.	Places call light and toilet tissue or wipes within resident's reach. Asks resident to clean hands with wipes if able. Asks resident to signal when finished and leaves room.		
18.	Discards disposable equipment. Cleans area.		
19.	Removes gloves and washes hands.		
20.	When called, returns and puts on clean gloves. Helps with perineal care as needed.		

Name: _____

21.	Removes bedpan. Removes bed protector.		
22.	Empties bedpan if used. Checks bedpan or toilet for consistency, color, and amount of stool.		
23.	Rinses bedpan and places in proper area for cleaning.		
24.	Removes and discards gloves		
25.	Washes hands.		
26.	Removes bath blanket. Returns bed to proper position.		
27.	Places call light within resident's reach.		
28.	Documents procedure.		

_____   _____
Date Reviewed   Instructor Signature

_____   _____
Date Performed   Instructor Signature

Collecting a stool specimen

	Procedure Steps	yes	no
1.	Washes hands.		
2.	Identifies self by name. Identifies resident by name.		
3.	Explains procedure to resident. Speaks clearly, slowly, and directly. Maintains face-to-face contact whenever possible.		
4.	Provides privacy.		
5.	Puts on gloves.		
6.	Asks resident not to urinate at the same time as moving bowels and not to put toilet paper in with the sample. Provides plastic bag to discard toilet paper separately.		
7.	Fits specimen pan to toilet or provides resident with bedpan. Leaves the room and asks the resident to call when he is finished. Makes sure call light is within reach.		

8.	When called, returns and helps as necessary with perineal care. Helps resident wash hands.		
9.	Removes and discards gloves.		
10.	Washes hands.		
11.	Puts on clean gloves.		
12.	Uses tongue blades to take about two tablespoons of stool and puts it in container without touching the inside. Covers container tightly. Places container in plastic bag.		
13.	Disposes of tongue blades and toilet paper. Empties bedpan or container into toilet. Rinses and takes to proper area for cleaning.		
14.	Removes and disposes of gloves.		
15.	Washes hands.		
16.	Returns bed to lowest position.		
17.	Places call light within resident's reach.		
18.	Takes specimen and lab slip to proper area. Documents procedure.		

_____   _____
Date Reviewed   Instructor Signature

_____   _____
Date Performed   Instructor Signature

Testing a stool specimen for occult blood

	Procedure Steps	yes	no
1.	Washes hands.		
2.	Puts on gloves.		
3.	Opens test card.		
4.	Gets small amount of stool from specimen container with tongue blade.		
5.	Smears small amount of stool onto Box A of test card.		

6.	Flips tongue blade and gets some stool from another part of specimen. Smears small amount of stool onto Box B of test card.		
7.	Closes test card and turns over to other side.		
8.	Opens the flap and opens developer. Applies developer to each box.		
9.	Waits the proper amount of time. Watches squares for color changes and records any changes.		
10.	Places tongue blade and test packet in plastic bag. Disposes of plastic bag properly.		
11.	Removes and discards gloves.		
12.	Washes hands.		
13.	Documents procedure.		

_____   _____
Date Reviewed   Instructor Signature

_____   _____
Date Performed   Instructor Signature

Caring for an ostomy

	Procedure Steps	yes	no
1.	Washes hands.		
2.	Identifies self by name. Identifies resident by name.		
3.	Explains procedure to resident, speaking clearly, slowly, and directly. Maintains face-to-face contact whenever possible.		
4.	Provides privacy.		
5.	Adjusts the bed to a safe working level, usually waist high. Locks bed wheels.		
6.	Places bed protector under resident. Covers resident with a bath blanket and only exposes the ostomy site. Offers resident a towel.		

7.	Puts on gloves.		
8.	Removes ostomy bag carefully and places it in plastic bag. Notes color, odor, consistency, and amount of stool in the bag.		
9.	Wipes area around the stoma with toilet paper or gauze. Discards paper/gauze in plastic bag.		
10.	Washes area around the stoma using a washcloth and warm soapy water. Moves in one direction, away from the stoma. Pats dry with another towel. Applies cream if ordered.		
11.	Places the clean ostomy appliance on resident, following instructions. Makes sure the bottom of the bag is clamped.		
12.	Removes disposable bed protector and discards. Places soiled linens in proper container.		
13.	Removes bag and bedpan and discards bag. Empties bedpan and rinses. Takes to proper area for cleaning.		
14.	Removes and discards gloves.		
15.	Washes hands.		
16.	Returns bed to lowest position.		
17.	Places call light within resident's reach.		
18.	Documents procedure.		

_____   _____
Date Reviewed   Instructor Signature

_____   _____
Date Performed   Instructor Signature

Putting elastic stockings on a resident

	Procedure Steps	yes	no
1.	Washes hands.		
2.	Identifies self by name. Identifies resident by name.		

Name: _____

	Procedure Steps	yes	no
3.	Explains procedure to resident, speaking clearly, slowly, and directly. Maintains face-to-face contact whenever possible.		
4.	Provides privacy.		
5.	With resident lying down, removes his or her socks, shoes, or slippers, and exposes one leg.		
6.	Turns stocking inside-out at least to heel area.		
7.	Gently places the foot of the stocking over toes, foot, and heel. Heel should be in right place (heel of foot should be in heel of stocking).		
8.	Gently pulls top of stocking over foot, heel, and leg.		
9.	Makes sure that there are no twists and wrinkles in the stocking after it is applied.		
10.	Repeats for the other leg.		
11.	Places call light within resident's reach.		
12.	Washes hands.		
13.	Documents procedure.		

_____   _____
Date Reviewed   Instructor Signature

_____   _____
Date Performed   Instructor Signature

Collecting a sputum specimen

	Procedure Steps	yes	no
1.	Washes hands.		
2.	Identifies self by name. Identifies resident by name.		
3.	Explains procedure to resident, speaking clearly, slowly, and directly. Maintains face-to-face contact whenever possible.		
4.	Provides privacy.		

	Procedure Steps	yes	no
5.	Puts on mask and gloves. Stands behind the resident if resident can hold container by himself.		
6.	Gives resident tissues to cover the mouth. Instructs resident to cough deeply and spit the sputum into the specimen container.		
7.	After sample has been obtained, covers container tightly, and wipes any sputum off the outside of the container. Puts container in plastic bag, and seals it.		
8.	Removes and discards gloves and mask.		
9.	Washes hands.		
10.	Places call light within resident's reach.		
11.	Documents procedure.		

_____   _____
Date Reviewed   Instructor Signature

_____   _____
Date Performed   Instructor Signature

Providing foot care for the diabetic resident

	Procedure Steps	yes	no
1.	Washes hands.		
2.	Identifies self by name. Identifies resident by name.		
3.	Explains procedure to resident, speaking clearly, slowly, and directly. Maintains face-to-face contact whenever possible.		
4.	Provides privacy.		
5.	Puts on gloves.		
6.	Washes feet with washcloth and soap, and rinses in warm water.		
7.	Pats the feet dry, wiping between the toes.		

8.	Gently rubs lotion into the feet with circular strokes. Does not put lotion in between the toes.		
9.	Observes the skin for signs of dryness, irritation, blisters, redness, sores, corns, discoloration, or swelling.		
10.	Assists resident with putting on socks and shoes or slippers.		
11.	Disposes of soiled linens in proper container and cleans and stores basin and supplies.		
12.	Removes and discards gloves.		
13.	Washes hands.		
14.	Places call light within resident's reach.		
15.	Documents procedure.		

_____ _____
Date Reviewed   Instructor Signature

_____ _____
Date Performed   Instructor Signature

21
Rehabilitation and Restorative Care

Assisting with passive range of motion exercises			
	Procedure Steps		
1.	Washes hands.		
2.	Identifies self by name. Identifies resident by name.		
3.	Explains procedure to resident, speaking clearly, slowly, and directly. Maintains face-to-face contact whenever possible.		
4.	Provides privacy.		
5.	Adjusts the bed to a safe working level, usually waist high. Locks bed wheels.		
6.	Positions resident in supine position.		
7.	Repeats each exercise at least three times.		

8.	**Shoulder:** Performs the following movements properly, supporting the resident's arm at the elbow and wrist by placing one hand under the elbow and the other hand under the wrist:		
	1. Flexion		
	2. Extension		
	3. Abduction		
	4. Adduction		
	Elbow: Performs the following movements properly, holding the wrist with one hand, and holding the elbow with the other:		
	1. Flexion		
	2. Extension		
	3. Pronation		
	4. Supination		
	Wrist: Performs the following movements properly, holding the wrist with one hand, and using the fingers of the other hand to help the joint through the motions:		
	1. Flexion		
	2. Extension		
	3. Radial flexion		
	4. Ulnar flexion		
	Thumb: Performs the following movements properly:		
	1. Abduction		
	2. Adduction		
	3. Opposition		
	4. Flexion		
	5. Extension		
	Fingers: Performs the following movements properly:		

200

Name: _____

	1. Flexion		
	2. Extension		
	3. Abduction		
	4. Adduction		
	Hip: Performs the following movements properly, placing one hand under the knee and one under the ankle:		
	1. Abduction		
	2. Adduction		
	3. Internal rotation		
	4. External rotation		
	Knees: Performs the following movements properly, placing one hand under the knee and one under the ankle:		
	1. Flexion		
	2. Extension		
	Ankles: Performs the following movements properly, supporting the foot and ankle:		
	1. Dorsiflexion		
	2. Plantar flexion		
	3. Supination		
	4. Pronation		
	Toes: Performs the following movements properly:		
	1. Flexion		
	2. Extension		
	3. Abduction		
	When all exercises are completed:		
9.	Returns resident to comfortable position and covers as appropriate. Returns bed to lowest position.		

10.	Places call light within resident's reach.		
11.	Washes hands.		
12.	Documents procedure. Notes any decrease in range of motion or any pain experienced by the resident. Notifies nurse if increased stiffness or physical resistance is noted.		

_____   _____
Date Reviewed   Instructor Signature

_____   _____
Date Performed   Instructor Signature

Practice Exam

Taking an Exam

After a nursing assistant has completed an approved training program in his or her state, he or she is given a competency evaluation (a certification exam or test) in order to be certified to work in that state. This exam usually consists of both a written evaluation and a skills evaluation. Here are some guidelines for taking exams so that you will be better prepared.

Your physical condition affects your mental abilities. Watch what you eat and drink before taking an exam and get plenty of rest. On the day of the exam, eat a healthy breakfast. It can be hard to think if you're hungry or if you did not eat a balanced breakfast. Also, being in good physical shape allows for more blood to get to your brain. A person who gets regular physical exercise has a body and mind that uses its oxygen more effectively than someone completely out of shape. Even exercising a few days before an exam can make a noticeable difference in your thinking powers.

When taking the exam, listen carefully to any instructions given. Be sure to read the directions. When taking a multiple choice test, first eliminate answers you know are wrong. Since your first choice is usually correct, do not change your answers unless you are sure of the correction. Do not spend too much time on any one question. If you do not understand it, move on and go back if time allows. Remember to leave that question blank on your answer sheet. Be careful to answer the next question in the proper space. For the skills portion of the exam, review the procedures in the book and any notes you may have taken.

Remember that being nervous is natural. Most people get nervous before and during a test. A little stress can actually help you focus and make you more alert. A few deep breaths can help calm you down. Try it. Most importantly, believe in yourself. You can do it!

1. When a resident refuses to let the nursing assistant take her blood pressure, the nursing assistant should
   (A) Tell the resident that she must have it taken to prevent a serious illness
   (B) Take the resident's blood pressure anyway
   (C) Tell the resident that if she does this, she will get a treat later
   (D) Report this to the nurse

2. A nursing assistant may share a resident's medical information with which of the following?
   (A) The resident's friends
   (B) Other members of the healthcare team
   (C) The nursing assistant's friends
   (D) The resident's roommate

3. To best communicate with a resident who has a hearing impairment, the nursing assistant should
   (A) Use short sentences and simple words
   (B) Shout
   (C) Approach the resident from behind
   (D) Raise the pitch of her voice

4. If a nursing assistant suspects that a resident is being abused, she should
   (A) Ask the resident if he thinks he is being abused
   (B) Call the resident's family and discuss the matter with them
   (C) Report it to the nurse immediately
   (D) Check with the resident's roommate to see if he has noticed anything

5. An ombudsman is a person who
   (A) Is in charge of the human resources department
   (B) Teaches nursing assistants how to perform ROM exercises
   (C) Is a legal advocate for residents and helps protect their rights
   (D) Creates special diets for residents

Name: _____

6. To best respond to a resident with Alzheimer's disease who is repeating a question over and over again, the nursing assistant should
   (A) Answer questions each time they are asked, using the same words
   (B) Try to silence the resident
   (C) Tell the resident to stop
   (D) Explain to the resident that he just asked that question

7. With regard to a resident's toenails, a nursing assistant should
   (A) Never cut them
   (B) Cut them when the resident requests it
   (C) Cut them daily
   (D) File them into rounded edges

8. When providing personal care, the nursing assistant should
   (A) Make sure the resident does not talk
   (B) Provide privacy for the resident
   (C) Tell the resident about other residents' conditions
   (D) Discuss personal problems

9. Generally, the last sense to leave a dying person is the sense of
   (A) Sight
   (B) Taste
   (C) Smell
   (D) Hearing

10. Which temperature site is considered the most accurate?
    (A) Rectal
    (B) Oral
    (C) Axillary
    (D) Tympanic

11. How should a standard bedpan be positioned?
    (A) According to the resident's preference
    (B) Wider end aligned with resident's buttocks
    (C) Smaller end aligned with resident's buttocks
    (D) Smaller end facing the resident's head

12. A resident tells a nursing assistant that she is scared of dying. How should the nursing assistant respond?
    (A) Reply, "You should attend church services more often. Then you probably won't be so afraid."
    (B) Listen quietly and ask questions when appropriate.
    (C) Tell the resident, "Don't worry so much. You won't be going anywhere soon."
    (D) Reply, "You need to start taking new medication."

13. To prevent dehydration, a nursing assistant should
    (A) Discourage fluids before bedtime
    (B) Withhold fluids so the resident will be really thirsty
    (C) Offer fresh water and other fluids often
    (D) Wake the resident during the night to offer fluids

14. When giving perineal care to a female resident, a nursing assistant should
    (A) Wipe from front to back
    (B) Wipe from back to front
    (C) Use the same section of the washcloth for cleaning each part
    (D) Wash the anal area before the perineal area

15. If a nursing assistant sees a resident masturbating, the nursing assistant should
    (A) Run to the charge nurse and ask her what to do
    (B) Provide privacy for the resident
    (C) Tell the resident that he should not be doing that
    (D) Tell the other nursing assistants what happened

16. In what order should range of motion exercises be done?
    (A) Start from the feet and work up
    (B) Start from the head and work down
    (C) The arms and legs should be exercised first
    (D) The arms and legs should be exercised last

17. A nursing assistant must wear gloves when
    (A) Combing a resident's hair
    (B) Feeding a resident
    (C) Performing oral care
    (D) Performing range of motion exercises

18. To best communicate with a resident who has a vision impairment, the nursing assistant should
    (A) Rearrange furniture without telling the resident
    (B) Identify herself when she enters the room
    (C) Keep the lighting low at all times
    (D) Touch the resident before identifying herself

19. The first sign of skin breakdown is:
    (A) Coolness
    (B) Bleeding
    (C) Discoloration
    (D) Numbness

20. Which one of the following statements is true of the normal aging process and late adulthood (65 years and older)?
    (A) People become helpless and lonely.
    (B) People become incontinent.
    (C) People develop Alzheimer's disease.
    (D) People are generally active and engaged.

21. Clean bed linens promote
    (A) Proper rest and sleep
    (B) Infection and disease
    (C) Pressure sores
    (D) Poor circulation

22. Abdominal thrusts help
    (A) Stop bleeding
    (B) Remove blockage from an airway
    (C) Reduce the risk of falls
    (D) Stop a heart attack

23. Which of the following is a way to prevent unintended weight loss?
    (A) Insisting that residents eat whatever food is offered to them
    (B) Hurrying residents through meals
    (C) Serving all residents the same food, regardless of likes and dislikes
    (D) Honoring food likes and dislikes

24. Which of the following is a way to use proper body mechanics while working?
    (A) Bending knees while lifting
    (B) Standing with feet close together while lifting
    (C) Holding objects far away from the body when carrying them
    (D) Twisting at the waist when moving an object

25. What would be the best way for a nursing assistant to promote a resident's independence and dignity during bowel or bladder retraining?
    (A) Rushing the resident
    (B) Providing privacy for elimination
    (C) Criticizing a resident when he has a setback
    (D) Withholding fluids

26. A resident tells a nursing assistant that he wants to wear his gray sweater. The nursing assistant should
    (A) Tell him that she has already picked out his clothes for the day
    (B) Tell him "OK" and assist him in getting dressed
    (C) Tell him that his gray sweater does not match his pants and ask him to pick something else
    (D) Tell him that she likes his blue sweater better

27. A nursing assistant should wash her hands
    (A) Only before a personal care procedure
    (B) Before and after a personal care procedure
    (C) Only after a personal care procedure
    (D) While wearing gloves

28. How should soiled bed linens be handled?
    (A) By carrying them away from the nursing assistant's body
    (B) By shaking them in the air to get rid of contaminants
    (C) By taking them into another resident's room
    (D) By taking them into the cafeteria

29. What is the purpose of the Health Insurance Portability and Accountability Act (HIPAA)?
    (A) To monitor quality of care in facilities
    (B) To reduce incidents of abuse in facilities
    (C) To keep protected health information private and secure
    (D) To provide training for facility staff

30. One safety device that helps transfer residents is called a
    (A) Waist restraint
    (B) Posey vest
    (C) Transfer belt
    (D) Geriatric chair

31. At which site is body temperature most often taken?
    (A) Armpit (axillary)
    (B) Ear (tympanic)
    (C) Mouth (oral)
    (D) Rectum (rectal)

32. A nursing assistant should encourage a resident's independence and self-care because doing this
    (A) Promotes body function
    (B) Decreases blood flow
    (C) Lowers self-esteem
    (D) Decreases the ability to sleep and rest

33. A restraint can be applied
    (A) When a resident is being rude
    (B) When a nursing assistant does not have time to watch the resident
    (C) With a doctor's order
    (D) When a resident keeps pressing his call light

34. A nursing assisting can show she is listening carefully to a resident by
    (A) Looking away when the resident talks
    (B) Changing the subject often
    (C) Rolling her eyes when the resident says something she doesn't agree with
    (D) Focusing on the resident and giving feedback

35. How many milliliters equal one ounce?
    (A) 40
    (B) 30
    (C) 60
    (D) 20

36. With catheters it is important for a nursing assistant to remember that
    (A) Tubing should be kinked
    (B) Perineal care does not need to be performed
    (C) The drainage bag should be kept lower than the hips or the bladder
    (D) The resident should lie on top of the tubing

37. When assisting a resident who has had a stroke, a nursing assistant should
    (A) Do everything for the resident
    (B) Lead with the stronger side when transferring
    (C) Dress the stronger side first
    (D) Place food in the affected, or weaker, side of the mouth

38. In which stage would a dying resident be if he insists that a mistake was made on his blood test and he's not really dying?
    (A) Denial
    (B) Bargaining
    (C) Acceptance
    (D) Depression

39. The process of helping to restore a person to the highest level of functioning is called
    (A) Positioning
    (B) Rehabilitation
    (C) Elimination
    (D) Retention

40. A nursing assistant overhears other nursing assistants discussing a resident. One of them says that she does not like taking care of this resident because "he is rude and smells funny." The nursing assistant should
    (A) Join in the conversation and tell the others her opinion of this resident
    (B) Let the resident know so that he will be nicer to the nursing assistants
    (C) Suggest to the nursing assistants that this isn't the place to have this discussion
    (D) Ask another resident's opinion of how she should respond

41. An oral temperature should not be taken on a resident who has eaten or had fluids in the last _____ minutes.
    (A) 25-35
    (B) 10-20
    (C) 40-50
    (D) 50-60

42. How many feet does a quad cane have?
    (A) 1
    (B) 2
    (C) 3
    (D) 4

43. A nursing assistant can assist residents with their spiritual needs by
    (A) Trying to convince residents to change to the nursing assistant's religion
    (B) Listening to residents talk about their beliefs
    (C) Insisting residents participate in religious services
    (D) Expressing judgments about residents' religious groups

44. The best way for a nursing assistant to respond to a combative resident is to
    (A) Hit the resident
    (B) Argue with the resident if what the resident is saying is wrong
    (C) Not take it personally
    (D) Let the resident know that he is behaving childishly

45. When a resident has a right-sided weakness, how should clothing be applied first?
    (A) On the left side
    (B) On the right side
    (C) On whichever side is closer to the nursing assistant
    (D) On whatever side the resident prefers

46. A resident offers a nursing assistant a gift for being such a good nursing assistant. The nursing assistant should
    (A) Politely refuse the gift
    (B) Politely accept the gift
    (C) Accept the gift but donate it to a homeless shelter
    (D) Tell the resident she would prefer money instead

47. According to OBRA, nursing assistants must complete at least ___ hours of training and must pass a competency evaluation before they can be employed.
    (A) 100
    (B) 250
    (C) 50
    (D) 75

48. Call lights should be placed
    (A) High on the wall over the head of the bed
    (B) Inside the bedside stand
    (C) On the floor
    (D) Within the resident's reach

49. How long should nursing assistants use friction when lathering and washing their hands?
    (A) 2 minutes
    (B) 5 seconds
    (C) 18 seconds
    (D) 20 seconds

50. The Occupational Safety and Health Administration (OSHA) is a federal government agency that protects workers from
    (A) Hazards on the job
    (B) Lawsuits
    (C) Workplace violence
    (D) Unfair employment practices

Name: _____